OXFORD MEDICAL PUBLI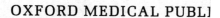

Obstetrics

Obstetrics
A Practical Manual

Roger Neuberg FRCOG

Consultant Obstetrician and Gynaecologist
Leicester Royal Infirmary
Leicester, UK

Oxford · New York · Tokyo
OXFORD UNIVERSITY PRESS
1995

Oxford University Press, Walton Street, Oxford OX2 6DP
Oxford   New York
Athens   Auckland   Bangkok   Bombay
Calcutta   Cape Town   Dar es Salaam   Delhi
Florence   Hong Kong   Istanbul   Karachi
Kuala Lumpur   Madras   Madrid   Melbourne
Mexico City   Nairobi   Paris   Singapore
Taipei   Tokyo   Toronto
and associated companies in
Berlin   Ibadan

Oxford is a trade mark of Oxford University Press

Published in the United States
by Oxford University Press Inc., New York

A catalogue record for this book is available from the British Library

Library of Congress Cataloging in Publication Data

Neuberg, Roger.
Obstetrics : a pratical manual / Roger Neuberg.
(Oxford medical publications)
Includes bibliographical references and index.
1. Obstetrics.   I. Title.   II. Series.
[DNLM: 1. Obstetrics.   2. Pregnancy.   3. Pregnancy Complications.
WQ 200 N478a 1995]
RG524.N49   1995   618.2 − dc20   94-34063

ISBN   0 19 263007 5

Typeset by Colset Private Limited, Singapore

Printed in Great Britain by Bookcraft (Bath) Ltd
Midsomer Norton, Avon

To all my junior colleagues, who keep me on my toes

Preface

I have written this book for the Senior House Officer, whether at the start of a career in obstetrics or in training for general practice, who has probably had no 'hands-on' experience since student days. I hope that midwives too will find it a useful addition to their already impressive list of reading material. The book may also be of interest to the undergraduate who is toying with the idea of coming back to the specialty after qualifying. Most obstetricians originally 'caught the bug' of this fascinating subject when, as medical students, they finally found out where babies came from!

It really is quite a daunting prospect for a non-academic like myself to dare to write a book for those in training. I have tried to give this book a different format and style from the usual type of training manual.

It would be impossible to cover the whole subject of obstetrics in 275 pages and that has never been my intention. There are already plenty of excellent standard textbooks available for that purpose. I have, however, tried to be as up-to-date as possible when it comes to the management of particular problems.

This book is intended to be a source of information dealing with the practical aspects of clinical work and not as a mini-textbook crammer giving all the essentials required to pass post-graduate examinations. It has been written in a logical chronological sequence from early pregnancy to the post-natal visit, to make reference easier. Simple line diagrams are used when required to clarify the text and there are clear boxed checklists on the important points to remember, especially when dealing with emergencies. Finally, there is a section which should be of practical help for those who will take the Diploma examination for the Royal College of Obstetricians and Gynaecologists.

It is important that the junior doctor should be able to adapt clinical practice to conform with the wishes of the consultant leading the team or those of the on-call consultant when there is an emergency problem. There may be management policies which will differ from the general guidelines given here. There will always be fine differences in management between specialists. I take full responsibility for my own!

Frequent reference is made in the text to the Report on Confidential Enquiries into Maternal Deaths. Familiarity with the Report by all obstetric and midwifery staff is, I believe, essential. Read it! Many maternal deaths have avoidable factors and one of the major factors is the lack of experience of the medical staff trying to cope with the emergency. To be aware of potential disaster does not imply a pre-occupation with gloom. Obstetrics is a very 'happy' specialty and I still get a kick from watching normal deliveries. But cautionary tales are useful.

Leicester   R. N.
January 1995

Acknowledgements

I am very grateful to my colleagues Paul Garrick and Farook Al-Azzawi for permitting me to reproduce Figures 2.8 and 3.1 respectively. I also thank Peter Gardiner for meticulously adapting his original illustrations produced above my text on episiotomy repair for GP Magazine (27/9/87). Barbara Wilson devoted much time to the typing of the tables used throughout the text and it is a pleasure to record my thanks to her.

The examination for the Diploma of the Royal College of Obstetricians & Gynaecologists (DRCOG) has dramatically changed its format from October 1994. I am indebted to Roger Jackson, Examination Secretary to the RCOG, for answering the many questions I put to him and especially for giving the time to check the accuracy of my chapter relating to the examination.

Finally I am very grateful for the amazing patience of the staff of Oxford University Press while awaiting the text of this book.

Contents

1   The diagnosis of pregnancy

It is very important to be able to diagnose pregnancy correctly. A woman will usually wish to have her suspicions, hopes, or fears confirmed one way or another as soon as possible. To assure a woman that she is not pregnant when in fact she is, or vice versa, can cause a considerable amount of distress and does not do a great deal to enhance a doctor's reputation. In the majority of cases the diagnosis of pregnancy is a simple matter, being based upon an assessment of symptoms and signs backed up by special investigations.

Symptoms and signs of early pregnancy

Symptoms

When a woman of reproductive age presents with amenorrhoea, having previously had a regular menstrual cycle, she should be regarded as being pregnant until proven otherwise. She can have any or all of the following symptoms: nausea, vomiting, excessive tiredness, increased breast fullness and tenderness, increased sensitivity and tingling around the nipples, and frequency of micturition. These symptoms together may be suggestive of a pregnancy but are not diagnostic.

Signs

On pelvic examination, owing to an increase in vascularity, the vagina and cervix have a purple–blue appearance rather than the non-pregnant pink hue. On bimanual palpation the uterus is enlarged and soft. The consistency of the pregnant cervix is rather like the softness of the lips of the mouth, whereas the non-pregnant cervix has a firmer consistency, more like the tip of the nose. It is common to feel arterial pulsation through each lateral fornix. When the uterus is palpated bimanually, it is usually quite easy to assess that it is enlarged in the early weeks, unless it is in a retroverted position. The uterine enlargement is often asymmetrical at this stage, as there is more pronounced uterine growth at the region of the placental site. There is no value in trying to elicit Hegar's sign. An undue amount of force may be applied while attempting to meet the fingers of the abdominal and vaginal hands through the softened and empty lower part of the uterus. At best this causes unnecessary discomfort and encourages a very real dread of future vaginal examinations, and at worst can cause vaginal bleeding and even miscarriage.

At 12 weeks gestation, the fundus of the uterus can be felt just above the symphysis pubis.

By the 12th week, breast signs will include primary pigmentation of the areola and nipples, prominence of Montgomery's tubercles in the areola, and an increased prominence of veins over the breasts.

Immunological pregnancy testing

The commercially available pregnancy testing kits depend upon the detection of human chorionic gonadotrophin (hCG) which has been secreted by the cells of the syncytiotrophoblast into the maternal circulation. Immunoassays have now been developed for the rapid and reliable detection of hCG. The commonly carried-out 'slide test' utilizes an agglutination–inhibition assay, whereby the hCG in an early-morning urine sample inhibits an agglutination reaction between hCG-coated latex particles and an antiserum. This type of immunoassay takes 2 minutes to perform and generally gives a positive result by day 42 (4 weeks after ovulation). The 2-hour test-tube version of this test, using hCG-coated red cells, is both more sensitive and more reliable, giving a positive result by day 36.

hCG is a glycoprotein consisting of two polypeptide sub-units, known as alpha and beta sub-units. Alpha sub-unit hCG is virtually identical to the alpha sub-units of luteinizing hormone (LH), follicle stimulating hormone (FSH) and thyroid stimulating hormone (TSH), so that antibodies to one will cross-react with the other. This can lead to false positive results. The detection of the beta sub-unit of hCG is specific for pregnancy and forms the basis of highly sensitive tests. Beta-hCG can be detected as early as 9 days after ovulation by enzyme-linked immunoassay using a monoclonal antibody. There is no cross-reaction with LH, FSH, or TSH. These immunospecific assays have been developed as rapid slide-tests to detect beta-hCG in urine, thereby allowing for the very early detection of pregnancy. However, the detection of beta-hCG in serum has the advantage of allowing serial quantitative measurements of hCG to be carried out. In practice this means that during the first 6 weeks of pregnancy the beta-hCG level doubles every 48 hours. Once the B-hCG level reaches 6000 IU/l, it should be possible to detect the pregnancy by ultrasonography.

A positive result is generally very reliable. There are now many kits on the market which can be bought as DIY kits by the general public. It must be remembered that cycles will vary in their lengths and that a negative test does not necessarily mean that a woman is not pregnant; the test may simply have been carried out too soon.

Ultrasound

Transabdominal ultrasonography can show the presence of a gestation sac as early as 6th week of pregnancy, and fetal heart movements can be detected during the 7th week. These scans can be difficult to assess especially if the maternal bladder is not full. The absence of fetal heart movements at this time does not necessarily imply that the pregnancy has come to grief. A repeat scan 1–2 weeks later will often pick up the fetal heart.

If ultrasonography is carried out using a vaginal probe, fetal heart movements can be recognized as early as 5 weeks. Vaginal ultrasound has the additional advantage of not requiring the patient to have a full bladder, a feature greatly appreciated by the recipient!

Symptoms and signs after the 12th week

Symptoms

Amenorrhoea, and breast heaviness and tenderness will be the persisting symptoms throughout pregnancy. Between the 12th and 16th weeks, nausea and vomiting should disappear, although these symptoms can persist for much longer. Frequency of micturition usually diminishes by the 12th week, only to reappear towards the end of pregnancy, due to the pressure of the presenting part of the baby upon the bladder. After the 12th week, the woman will begin to notice an increase in abdominal girth and be able to feel a swelling in the lower abdomen. The abdominal swelling enlarges progressively. The primigravida will usually first notice fetal movements (quickening) by the 18th–20th week whereas the multiparous woman who has learned from previous experience how to recognize movements will tend to feel these 2 weeks earlier. This is a generalization with very wide variation. Some women find it impossible to feel movements at all.

As the pregnancy progress, the uterus gradually fills the abdomen, often producing considerable discomfort, shortness of breath, and difficulty in walking. In primigravidae the upper abdominal discomfort is often relieved after the 36th week (lightening), owing to the descent of the presenting part of the baby into the pelvis. In the later weeks of pregnancy, painless tightenings (Braxton Hicks contractions) of the uterus can be felt.

Signs

By the 16th week, it is possible to express colostrum from the breasts, and by mid-pregnancy there is often additional pigmentation around the primary areola (known as secondary areola). There is also an increase in pigmentation of any scars, the appearance of the linea nigra extending downwards from the umbilicus, and often a blotchy pigmentation over the face, especially the cheeks and forehead (chloasma uterinum). A proportion of women will develop stretch marks (striae gravidarum) which are reddish in colour. Older striae, whether due to obesity or from a previous pregnancy, have a silvery appearance.

The major feature of the last three-quarters of pregnancy is the increasing size of the uterus. After the 12th week the fundus of the uterus is palpable above the symphysis pubis. Fig. 1.1 is a familiar picture but at best is purely a guide.

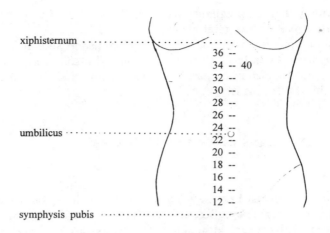

Fig. 1.1   Diagram of fundal height/weeks of pregnancy.

It is, in fact, quite unusual to find the 'standard umbilicus' conveniently sited at 22–24 weeks. The height and stature of the patient, the presence of obesity, or even just very tense abdominal muscles, lead to considerable variability in the site of the umbilicus. Furthermore, the xiphisternum is also a movable feast and in the very tall patient the fundus of the uterus will never reach it. The only relatively stable feature is the symphysis pubis. With experience, the clinician is able to assess uterine size reasonably accurately by palpation. There is also a good correlation between the period of gestation and the height in centimetres from the top of the symphysis up to the fundus of the uterus. So at 24 weeks, the syphysis-to-fundus height will be approximately 24 cm and at 36 weeks 36 cm. By measuring the fundal height in this way, the majority of babies that are going to become 'small-for-dates' will be detected. After 36 weeks, measuring the fundal height becomes less accurate, owing to engagement of the presenting part that can occur at this time and the variability in the size of babies. Thus, a 3 kg baby at term, can be the same size as a 36-week baby that will finally weigh 4 kg at term. Measuring the abdominal girth is less accurate, being approximately 24 inches at 24 weeks, and increasing by an inch per week to reach 40 inches at term. Adjustments would need to be made for the fatter or thinner patient.

By 24–26 weeks it is usually possible to recognize fetal parts, and ballottement of the head can be elicited. There is little point in determining the lie, presentation, and position of the fetus until after 30 weeks.

From the 12th week, the fetal heart can be picked up by ultrasound using an external transducer. In the very thin woman it may be possible to hear the fetal heart using a Pinard stethoscope after the 21st week, but it is more usual to find this sign after 24 weeks. The fetal heart is most clearly heard through the upper fetal back and varies between 120 and 160 beats per minute. If the woman's wrist is held at the same time, it is easy to distinguish the slower maternal pulse rate from the more rapid fetal heart rate. In time with the maternal pulse rate is the uterine souffle which is the soft blowing sound made by the increased blood flow through the uterus. The funic souffle is a soft sound of similar quality but in time with the fetal heart rate, and is due to blood flow through the umbilical cord.

X-ray diagnosis of pregnancy is now only rarely carried out owing to the general availability of ultrasound. There is still a place for X-rays later in pregnancy when certain types of fetal abnormality are suspected, or to confirm the number of fetuses in a known multiple pregnancy.

Pseudocyesis

A prolonged stressful disturbance such as an overwhelming desire to have a baby, or any other major emotional crisis, can produce all of the symptoms and many of the signs of pregnancy. These women will have amenorrhoea, breast symptoms, secretion of fluid from the nipples, and abdominal distension whether from fat or air swallowing. They can convince themselves and sometimes their medical attendants that they are indeed pregnant. The movement of flatus in the bowel is interpreted as fetal movement. Pelvic examination may be difficult to interpret especially in the early weeks of the 'pregnancy'. Once it becomes obvious that there is no uterine enlargement, ultrasonography and pregnancy testing reveal the true state of affairs. Sometimes these women will insist that they are pregnant in the face of all the evidence and may visit one doctor after another to try to get support for their own diagnosis. Great tact and sympathy is required in caring for these women. A psychiatric referral may also be necessary.

Differential diagnosis of a large abdominal swelling

A smooth swelling of the abdomen is not always due to a pregnancy. The differential diagnosis will include the following six 'f's: fetus, fat, fluid (in an ovarian cyst, full bladder, or ascites), fibroid, flatus, and faeces (the world record for constipation is one year!).

A summary of the symptoms and signs of pregnancy is given in Table 1.1.

Table 1.1   Summary of symptoms and signs of pregnancy

Symptoms	Weeks	Signs
Amenorrhoea	4	**+ve beta-hCG pregnancy test**
Nausea/vomiting > tiredness		Uterine changes
Breast fullness/sensitivity		**FH seen on ultrasound scan**
Frequency of micturition	8	Vaginal and cervical changes Early breast signs
	12	Uterus palpable abdominally **FH heard with ultrasound** (Progressive uterine growth)
'Quickening', (multipara)	16	Colostrum can be expressed
'Quickening' (primigravida)	20	Secondary areola
Braxton Hicks contractions	24	**Ballottement of fetal parts** **FH heard on auscultation**
	28	**Visible fetal movements** **Fetus can be clearly** **seen on X-ray**
	32	
'Lightening'	36	Descent of presenting part in the primigravida
	40	

Signs in **bold underlined** lettering are the only absolute diagnostic signs of pregnancy.

There are no absolute diagnostic symptoms of pregnancy. *Every* symptom of pregnancy can occur in pseudocyesis.

Timing of symptoms and non-underlined signs can be very variable.

2   Antenatal care

There is no doubt that it is more dangerous for a woman to be pregnant than non-pregnant. Therefore, the aim of antenatal care must be to ensure that she emerges from pregnancy safely and has a happy outcome in the form of a live and healthy baby. How can this desirable result be achieved?

(1) Appropriate pre-conception counselling;

(2) early booking for antenatal care;

(3) keeping the woman and her partner well-informed about pregnancy, dispelling any myths and fears they may have about labour, and preparing them for the eventual care of their baby;

(4) screening to detect fetal abnormality;

(5) detection and treatment of complications of pregnancy;

(6) monitoring of fetal well-being;

(7) detection of possible labour problems before labour commences, e.g. cephalo-pelvic disproportion;

(8) delivery in the safest environment.

Pre-conception counselling

Good antenatal care begins before pregnancy. It is in every woman's interests that she embarks upon pregnancy as fit and as healthy as possible and has done everything possible to ensure a happy outcome. Ideally, every woman should seek the advice of a health care professional *before* her first pregnancy. Pre-conception counselling, whether by the general practitioner, family planning clinic, health visitor, community midwife, or a hospital clinic may improve both morbidity and mortality rates.

There are particular woman groups who should seek advice:

(1) The nulliparous woman;

(2) the infertile couple;

(3) where there is an existing medical condition, such as diabetes, heart disease, epilepsy and other disorders where regular medication is required, e.g. steroids for asthmatics;

(4) where there is a family history of inherited disorders;

(5) following miscarriage, stillbirth, or neonatal death;

(6) following a fetal abnormality;

(7) where there is a very complex past obstetric history.

A full history is taken and an examination is carried out. Urine is tested for sugar and protein. A full blood count is taken as well as screening for rubella immunity. It is not sufficient to simply rely upon a past history of having had rubella or even upon vaccination as a schoolgirl, since at least 5 per cent of vaccines fail to give immunity.

General counselling will include advice on diet, alcohol, and cigarette smoking, so there may be a need for the woman to adjust her lifestyle to quite a major degree. There may be a need to discuss the timing of pregnancy, especially if there are investigations planned for other medical problems, such as intravenous urography. Advice on contraception may be more appropriate while her medical problems are being sorted out. If a surgical procedure is being considered for any condition, should it be performed before a pregnancy or be deferred? Will pregnancy affect any benefit gained by surgery? Will an operation affect the management of a subsequent pregnancy? An example of these two problems is seen in the woman who elects to have her operation for stress incontinence of urine carried out before her family is complete. If the operation is successful, there is the possibility that merely by being pregnant her incontinence will return. If, on the other hand, she remains dry during her subsequent pregnancy, it may be best to protect the operation by means of a Caesarean section, rather than to allow the pressure and stretching that occurs during a vaginal delivery possibly to undo the good results of the surgery.

The older woman needs careful advice so that she appreciates the problems she may face in a pregnancy, as well as the decisions she may need to take on screening tests for Down's syndrome. The infertile couple, or the woman who had had recurrent miscarriages, may require referral to the infertility clinic. Where there are known pre-existing medical conditions it may be necessary to refer to an appropriate specialist to obtain the 'all clear' before she even attempts to become pregnant. Drug therapy may need to modified.

In an attempt to prevent the *first occurrence* of a neural tube defect, it is recommended that all women who are planning a pregnancy should take a daily dietary supplement of 0.4 mg of folic acid, either alone or included in a supplement of B group vitamins. If there has been a past history of a neural tube defect, the minimum daily recommended supplement of folic acid is 5 mg. The folic acid preparation is continued throughout the first 12 weeks of pregnancy.

An obstetrician is the best person to advise upon the significance of past obstetric problems and the bearing that these may have upon a woman's future pregnancy. A plan of management in that pregnancy can then be outlined. She will also be alerted to the importance of early antenatal booking.

The services of a clinical geneticist are invaluable when there is a family history of hereditary disorders, or where there has been the loss of a baby due to a congenital abnormality. Obviously the couple's chief concern will be the answers to the questions 'Why did it happen and will it happen again?'

As a result of pre-conception counselling, a woman should be able to ensure that both she and her partner are fit and healthy when she does conceive and that she has done everything possible to improve her prospects of a happy outcome.

Place of confinement

The majority of women will follow the advice of their medical carers regarding the best place to have their baby. The choices include the *consultant unit, midwife-run unit, GP unit*, and *home confinement*.

Labour is generally acknowledged to be an intensive care situation, where potentially life-threatening problems for the mother or baby can arise with extraordinary rapidity. On that basis, many women and obstetricians are convinced that the consultant unit must be the safest place for a woman to be when in labour. The concept of 'team midwifery' means that a team of midwives are linked to each consultant and will care for that consultant's patients in antenatal clinics, on the ward, and on the labour ward. This gives continuity of care for the woman, who has the opportunity of building up a relationship with the nursing staff she will meet on admission.

However, there can be no doubt that many midwives have great skills which are considerably under-utilized. A well-trained midwife is completely capable of carrying out routine antenatal care herself, and of managing the progress of normal labour without any medical intervention whatsoever. Gradually, more 'midwife-run' units are being established. All of these are linked to a consultant unit and most of them are actually within the same establishment. These units have very clear guidelines as to when to seek medical assistance, be it antenatally or in labour. A specialized 'home from home' unit where the delivery rooms are designed like normal bedrooms will also appeal to the woman who wishes to have a normal 'low tech' labour and yet have the reassurance that expert help is just down the corridor if required.

Throughout the country there are excellent GP units which can undertake normal deliveries; delivery is conducted by the woman's own community midwife and general practitioner. Some of these GP units are able to deliver their patients within the consultant unit labour ward which is ideal, as there is rapid access to both specialist obstetric and paediatric facilities. Those GP units which serve more remote rural areas are obviously going to be further away from specialist assistance. The majority of such units have become very skilled at predicting problems before they occur and will readily transfer patients to the consultant unit.

For the very low-risk woman a domiciliary delivery may be considered. This will be carried out by the community midwife with the back-up of the woman's medical practitioner and the 'flying squad' if required. Some women and their partners will forcefully put the case for a home confinement even when there are definite medical contraindications, and will persist in their demands in spite of any well-reasoned medical objection. It is worth while to attempt to reach a compromise in such cases, such as delivery in the consultant unit and same-day discharge home. If there is a 'home from home' unit, this may appeal as an alternative arrangement. There is, however, little point in having a battle on the issue — care in labour must be provided regardless. The medical records must be clearly documented with the information that the woman has been fully informed of the risks she is taking and that she is acting against medical advice. Her general practitioner must also be informed.

Antenatal care is usually carried out in one of the following ways:

1. *Shared antenatal care.* This is the most common form of antenatal care where delivery is planned for the consultant unit. The number of attendances at the hospital will vary but, when everything is straightforward, will generally include a booking visit, and antenatal attendances at 28 weeks, 36 weeks, term, and thereafter until delivery. The GP and community midwife will undertake the remainder of the antenatal care. The advantages of shared care are that it takes the pressure off large, busy, specialist clinics, and it is often more convenient for the woman to see her GP. It also allows her to get to know her midwife who will, after all, be looking after her when she returns home with the baby.

2. *Total consultant unit care.* This is indicated in the high-risk pregnancy, where there is likely to be a major antenatal problem, requiring close monitoring. These patients are likely to require antenatal admission.

3. *GP and community midwife care.* The consultant unit is generally not involved in antenatal care when delivery is planned for either the GP unit or the woman's own home. There may, however, be an initial request for consultant unit assessment for suitability for one of these two options. These women will only be referred back to the consultant unit should a problem arise either antenatally or in labour.

The following woman categories are generally accepted as requiring consultant unit booking for delivery:

- *all primigravidae*, particularly the very young, the 'elderly' over the age of 30, those of small stature, where there has been a history of infertility;
- *multiparous women having their 5th or subsequent labour;*
- *where there are pre-existing medical conditions*, e.g. diabetes, essential hypertension, cardiac disease;
- *where there have been obstetric problems in a previous pregnancy*, e.g. hypertension, APH, intrauterine growth retardation (IUGR), premature labour, precipitate or prolonged labour, difficult forceps delivery, Caesarean section, *any* third stage of labour problem, third-degree tear, fetal abnormality, intrauterine death, neonatal death, problems of the puerperium;
- *where there is a problem in the current pregnancy*, e.g. unknown dates, anaemia, APH, multiple pregnancy, pregnancy-induced hypertension, rhesus iso-immunization, IUGR, unstable lie, and other problems that were not apparent at booking.

The antenatal booking appointment

The timing of the booking appointment at the antenatal clinic is variable, but is usually before the 12th week. During this visit, a history is taken and an examination is carried out. The full booking blood tests may be taken at this visit unless already done by the GP. To save the woman a pin-prick some clinics will defer the routine blood tests until the 15th week when it may be planned to take blood for prenatal screening. An early-morning urine sample is tested. Frequently an ultrasound scan is carried out at this attendance.

The history

There is considerable variation in records from one hospital to another, although it is hoped that there will eventually be standardization of maternity notes. The history falls into the following sections:

1. Social history. The woman's personal and social details are taken. Her address and contact telephone numbers are obviously important, as are those of her GP and community midwife.

It is relevant to enquire into her marital status, the stability of her relationship with her partner, and her general home situation. This will help to determine the amount of support she will be receiving from him and may indicate an early referral to the clinic's medical social worker. The single unsupported woman or schoolgirl may have very great social problems.

Her occupation is noted. Enquiry is made into her diet (e.g. is she vegetarian?). Information about her lifestyle, including details of smoking, alcohol intake, regular medications, and any drug allergies is recorded.

2. Past medical history. Enquiry should be made into all past medical problems and operations. If there is no obtainable past medical history, it is worth while to ask if she has ever been admitted to hospital for *anything* at all. What may have seemed minor and trivial to the woman may be of considerable relevance in the context of a pregnancy. A history of a past blood transfusion is important.

3. Past family history. It can be very helpful to have details of the past and current health of the patient's family, since potential problems that may be relevant to the pregnancy can be highlighted. This is especially true when there is a past history of diabetes and hypertension. If this information is not volunteered by the woman, she should be directly asked about these two conditions. A family history of TB should be sought from any woman from the Asian sub-continent. A history of multiple pregnancy on either side of the family is relevant.

It is important tactfully to ask if any children have been born into the family who have a physical or mental disability or handicap.

4. Past obstetric history. Every pregnancy is documented in chronological

PAST OBSTETRIC HISTORY							Grav. **4**		Para **2**		Children alive **2**	
Date	Place	Durat (wks)	Antenatal complic.	S I	Durat labour (hrs)	Method of Del.	3rd stage	Puerperium	Sex	Wt. (kg.)	Fetal outcome Feeding
1987	LRI	11	Missed Abortion. ERPC								
1988	LRI	41	None	S	3	Emergency LSCS (fetal distress)			M	3.99	A&W (Br.)
						2⊙ transfused to replace op. loss					
1991	LRI	38	Amniocentesis			Elective LSCS			F	4.09	A&W (Br.)

Fig. 2.1   Example of recording of obstetric history.

order, noting the year, place of confinement, any antenatal problems, the duration of pregnancy, whether labour was induced or had a spontaneous onset, the duration of labour, the method of delivery, any third stage problems, or problems in the puerperium. The weight, sex, health, and method of feeding of the baby are also recorded. (See Fig. 2.1.)

5. *Current pregnancy history.* It is worthwhile asking if this pregnancy is a planned one, a happy—or indeed unhappy—accident. Significant details can become apparent that may otherwise be missed in taking the routine social history. Details of previous contraception should also be noted.

If obstetricians have an obsession over anything it is over dates! Although ultrasound can solve many date problems and can clarify the situation, a carefully taken menstrual history can be invaluable.

When enquiring about the date of the woman's last normal menstrual period (LMP), the reliability of that date is essential when it comes to calculating the expected date of delivery (EDD). There are several back-up questions that can help to determine the normality of that period:

- 'How regular were your periods and for how many days did they normally last?'
- 'Did the last period come when it was expected?'
- 'Did it last the normal length of time?'
- 'Were you on the Pill immediately before the last period?' (was it a Pill-withdrawal bleed?)
- 'Have you had any bleeding since your last period?'

Having established the reliability of the LMP, it is then simple to calculate the EDD, by adding 7 days to the day of the month and then either adding 9 to the month or subtracting 3:

e.g. LMP 11th March 1995 . . . . EDD 18th December 1995
LMP 28th November 1994 . . . . . EDD 5th September 1995

However, if the cycle length is erratic, e.g. periods occurring every 6–8 weeks, the EDD will probably be 2–4 weeks later than the date calculated by the above method. Confirmation of the date is obtained by a combination of clinical examination to determine the size of the uterus and ultrasound measurement of the fetus. It is important that patients with uncertain dates or an irregular cycle are referred early so that there is at least an opportunity to sort out a reliable EDD. If the EDD remains vague, it becomes more difficult to recognize fetal growth retardation. Problems will also arise over the question of postmaturity when an unreliable EDD is reached. It is interesting that less than 5 per cent of womans actually deliver on their due date. There is a growing move to give patients a range of dates when it is likely that they will deliver, i.e. from 38th to 42nd weeks. This would in fact reassure many women with normal pregnancies who understandably become concerned when they 'go past their dates'.

A history of the pregnancy to date is now taken with regard to assessing the woman's general well-being and state of health. Enquiry should be made after symptoms of nauseas vomiting, and any medications that she may be taking for these symptoms or for any other problem. There may be a specific line of questioning that will have been indicated by some feature of her past medical history. The planned method of feeding the baby is recorded.

Booking examination

A general physical examination is carried out. This will include:

- measurement of height
- weight (kg)
- breast examination
- cardiovascular system
- respiratory system.

The abdomen is palpated. The uterus will usually only be palpable above the symphysis pubis at 12 weeks (Fig. 1.1). As with any mass rising up out of the pelvis, it is important to come down onto the mass with the examining hand starting in the upper abdomen. It is otherwise surprisingly easy to miss the fundus of the uterus if the palpation is made only in the lower abdomen.

Before the routine availability of ultrasound, a pelvic examination as part of the first booking examination was invaluable. Now it is often argued that if an ultrasound scan has been taken at the booking visit, it is no longer necessary to perform a pelvic examination. However, while a scan may give accurate information regarding the gestational age of the fetus, it is still of value to know the clinical size of the uterus at booking. It is not uncommon later in pregnancy, when there may be some date/size/scan discrepancy, to rely quite heavily on the initial bimanual assessment made by an experienced clinician. There is no doubt that the information gained from a reliable vaginal examination is of more clinical value than an unreliable ultrasound, e.g. when the bladder is not full.

The following findings will be detected on vaginal examination, but could be missed on scan:

(1) vaginal septum;

(2) patulous cervix (which may become incompetent);

(3) cervical pathology (ectopy, polypi, carcinoma);

(4) bicornuate uterus;

(5) acutely retroverted uterus (which could become impacted at 15 weeks).

An initial impression of the size and shape of the pelvis is also obtained, although this is not the time to fully assess the pelvic capacity.

Before a vaginal examination is carried out on a pregnant woman it is essential to reassure her that internal examinations do not cause miscarriages. Many women are understandably apprehensive of either being hurt or of losing their pregnancy as a result of such an examination. Some will also find it intensely embarrassing. It is important to be sensitive to these worries and feelings. A very gentle vaginal examination, with the lower abdomen and upper thighs draped, will reveal much more information than a vigorous one which will only result in abdominal and pelvic muscle rigidity and a reluctance to permit any similar examinations in the future. If the pregnancy has been unstable in the early weeks, e.g. a major threat to miscarry, then it is best to defer the examination.

If she has not had a cervical smear in the previous 18 months, it is reasonable to take an opportunistic smear at the booking examination.

Early ultrasound scan

All consultant unit antenatal clinics will have an ultrasound service. It is very useful to be able to have the results of an ultrasound scan available at the booking visit. The scan will be able to give a considerable amount of valuable information. Furthermore, the majority of patients will know something about ultrasound and will often request a scan if not offered one as part of the routine assessment. Apart from being of intense interest to the couple, it is also immensely reassuring and a very significant experience for them.

The benefits of early ultrasound are:

- confirmation of an ongoing pregnancy
- early detection of hydatidiform mole
- scan dating (? compatible with actual calendar dates) by accurately measuring the crown–rump length between the 7th and 12th weeks
- initial placental localization
- diagnosis of multiple pregnancy
- early diagnosis of some major abnormalities.

The findings at the initial scan may indicate a need for repeat scans later in the pregnancy. For example, a low-lying placenta found early in pregnancy may, by the third trimester, have been drawn out of the 'danger zone' which will form the lower segment of the uterus. However, the chance finding of such a placental site at routine scanning will alert the obstetrician to repeat placental localization at 28–32 weeks. (The patient will also be warned to report any vaginal blood loss immediately. She should be advised not to indulge in too vigorous intercourse with deep penetration.) It should also be stressed that scans in the first trimester are unable to exclude a number of abnormalities of the fetus which might only be detectable by 'detailed scanning' between 18 and 22 weeks (p. 36). Some clinics are able to offer such scanning as a routine screen.

Booking investigations

The routine booking investigations will include:

(1) full blood count;

(2) blood group (if rhesus-negative, antibody screening);

(3) hepatitis B (Australia antigen) screening;

(4) rubella antibody screening;

(5) serological screening for syphilis (TPHA, VDRL);

(6) mid-stream urine for culture;

(7) urine testing for protein and glucose;

(8) electrophoresis to screen for beta-thalassaemia among women of Mediterranean origin and from the Asian subcontinent;

(9) sickle-cell screen on all Afro-Caribbean patients.

A chest X-ray is no longer a routine antenatal investigation. It is, however, worth while to consider screening immigrant patients for TB, especially those who have recently arrived from the Asian subcontinent.

(If there is a need for prenatal diagnosis, it is usually discussed at the time of the booking appointment. This very important subject is considered at the end of this chapter.)

General advice to the patient

Once the woman has had her pregnancy confirmed by her own GP, it is likely that she will have received some general advice about care of herself during the early weeks of pregnancy. Usually this will have been on the lines of using 'common sense' and to avoid excesses of physical activity, especially at the times when she would have had a period had she not been pregnant.

Antenatal clinics can provide beautifully illustrated and informative booklets on all aspects of pregnancy. Clinics run classes and discussion groups (which the woman should encourage her partner to attend) which give the hospital staff an ideal opportunity to allay the fears that many women have about pregnancy in general and labour in particular. Guided tours of different parts of the hospital including antenatal and postnatal wards, the labour ward itself, and the special care baby unit, help to familiarize the woman with the hospital environment and do much to reduce anxiety when the time comes for her own admission.

Relaxation classes can teach her to cope better with the pain of labour. Information on pain relief, the availability of TENS (Transdermal Electrical Nerve Stimulation) units, and epidurals in particular, should be offered to the patient. It should be stressed that a request for an epidural does not mean that she has in any way failed or let herself down. In fact, the knowledge that there is an epidural service available an request can do much to reassure the apprehensive patient.

Parentcraft classes can be a useful introduction prior to actually handling and looking after a baby.

The booking appointment is also a suitable time for the clinic midwife and doctor to give the woman additional guidance regarding her health and lifestyle during the pregnancy.

Diet

Common-sense advice on a correct balanced diet is available to all pregnant women in antenatal clinics. During pregnancy a daily calorie intake of 2500 kcal is advisable. A good variety of foods is important, with the protein content increasing in the last trimester. Vegetarians may find this more difficult to do. Most clinics have the services of a dietician available should difficulties arise.

In recent years, there has been a whole range of advice an what may or may not be safe for a pregnant woman to eat. The most recent 'scares' have been that paté and soft ripened cheeses may predispose to listeriosis, and that a high intake of vitamin A may lead to birth defects. Vitamin A is essential for normal good health and pregnant women have traditionally been advised to make sure that they receive enough of this in their diet. However, the Department of Health has now advised that pregnant women should not eat liver or liver products as the high levels of vitamin A they contain may be harmful to the fetus.

Alcohol

It has been traditional to advise all pregnant women to abstain from alcohol. However, no correlation has been found between a low alcohol intake (less than 8 units or 120 g per week) and fetal abnormality. A high alcohol intake (above 200 g per week), especially during the first trimester, is associated with abortion, intrauterine growth retardation, central nervous system abnormalities which include microcephaly, facial deformities, hypotonia, behavioural problems, mental retardation ('fetal alcohol syndrome'), and delayed infant development.

Smoking

The risks of smoking in pregnancy are proven. It has been calculated that 8000 pregnancies are lost each year in the UK as a direct consequence of cigarette smoking. The risk of abortion is 30–70 per cent higher among smoking women and increases with the number of cigarettes smoked each day. There is also an increased risk of premature labour and a higher perinatal mortality rate. These babies tend to be small for dates and this growth retardation can continue into infancy. It has been shown that carbon monoxide levels in fetal blood are 2.5 times higher than in maternal blood. This is really implying that if a woman is smoking 20 cigarettes a day, her baby is being forced to 'smoke' 50. It should be explained to the woman that as she will be taking most of the oxygen supply in her blood for herself, the baby gets only a small amount; and, if what little oxygen that is left for her baby cannot combine with the baby's own haemoglobin because it has already combined with carbon monoxide from smoking, the danger in which she is putting her baby may be appreciated. Nobody can pretend that to give up an addiction that may have been enjoyed in the past is easy. It is important to use a sympathetic approach but also to make quite certain that she understands the risks of smoking and not to play these down. Many women will be highly motivated to stop and it may also be an opportunity for their partners to stop smoking too.

Work

If the woman's occupation is not too strenuous, there is no reason why she should not continue to work until the end of the second trimester and perhaps beyond that date. However, very major physical effort should be avoided. A man should not forget that housework comes into this category, such as dragging the vacuum cleaner upstairs, moving the beds, etc. During the later weeks, it is important that she is able to literally put her feet up and rest for at least 2 hours each afternoon. If the pregnancy has been unstable in the early weeks with threats to miscarry, or if there is a past history of previous pregnancy losses, it may be advisable to stop work sooner.

Exercise

Most women are healthier in pregnancy than they are at any other time in their lives. There is no reason to curtail normal exercise such as walking and swimming. (Probably at 38 weeks swimming in the local swimming pool should stop, just in case she ruptures her membranes spontaneously and the whole pool has to be drained!) She may feel fit enough to continue with sporting activities such as horse-riding, but feeding the horse sugar lumps is safer. Major problems may arise if she should fall off; the same advice applies to cycling and skiing.

Travel

Women will frequently ask if it is all right to travel abroad when pregnant. The actual mechanics of travel in modern pressurized aircraft do not present a problem. However, in the event of miscarriage or any other obstetric complication, she is going to be out of her normal environment, may not speak the language, and may not have available the full emergency facilities that she would have had, had she stayed at home. Therefore, the counsel of perfection would be to advise that she has her holiday somewhere in the home country, because in an emergency, any treatment that she receives, whether in Bournemouth, Leicester, or Glasgow will be very similar. If she does decide to travel abroad, she should avoid the first trimester when the miscarriage risk is greater and the last 8 weeks when the airline may refuse to bring her back! She should take out separate insurance to cover her for any problems that may occur relating to the pregnancy. She should only drink water that has been bottled and avoid any exotic food with which she is unfamilar.

Ideally, vaccination should be avoided whenever possible, unless the woman will be at greater risk without the vaccine. Malaria prophylaxis will be required if she must travel to an area where malaria is endemic. It is possible to find out from the local Drug Information Service, the type of malaria that is endemic in the region to which travel is proposed, and the best prophylaxis that can be used.

Sexual intercourse

Intercourse can take place at any time in a normal pregnancy. In fact many women find that they gain more pleasure from a loving relationship during pregnancy than at other times in their lives. The increasing abdominal girth can lead to some difficulties with access, but it can be fun adapting to other positions. If there has been a history of miscarriages, it would make sense to abstain during the first trimester. Intercourse does not lead to miscarriage, but abstention under these circumstances will avoid feelings of guilt should another miscarriage occur. If there has actually been bleeding during the pregnancy, or it is known that the placenta is low-lying during the second trimester, then intercourse with deep penetration should be avoided.

Breast care

A decision to breast-feed should be encouraged whenever possible, but it is pointless to attempt coercion. If the woman does decide against breast-feeding, breast care advice is appreciated even if just for cosmetic reasons. Pregnant women should be advised to wear a bra that gives good support rather than being merely decorative. Stretch marks over the breasts might be upsetting, and are to some degree avoidable if support is adequate. She should also consider wearing a 'sleep bra' at night. If she is planning to breast-feed her baby, she should be advised on preparing the nipples especially if they have been found to be inverted. Massage of the nipples or occasionally the wearing of Waller shells within the bra can help the nipples to evert. From 30 weeks the breasts can be further prepared by teaching her to massage them towards the nipple and express colostrum. A failure to do this can lead to milk duct obstruction.

Dental care

Every woman should attend her dentist during pregnancy. Gum disorders are common and can be kept under control with correct advice and treatment. Treatment is free for the duration of the pregnancy and the following year.

Drugs in pregnancy

Ever since the thalidomide tragedy, there has been understandable caution over any medication used in pregnancy, especially during the first trimester when organogenesis is taking place. Not only are the doctor and pharmacist wary, but many women themselves are hesitant over taking any drugs at all during pregnancy or while breast-feeding. It is right and proper that pregnant women should query their prescriptions. The medical profession should welcome their concern and not take offence if it seems that their professional judgement is being questioned. The data sheets for most drugs will carry one of the following well-recognized statements:

Safety for use in pregnancy has not been established.

Do not use in pregnancy/lactation unless there are compelling reasons.

Do not use in early pregnancy, unless in the judgement of the physician the potential benefits outweigh the risks.

Animal teratology and reproduction studies have demonstrated no adverse effects. However, as with all drugs, caution is recommended when used in early pregnancy.

It must be remembered that, with the exception of heparin, virtually all drugs will cross the placental barrier. When drugs *are* prescibed in pregnancy, whenever possible well-tried preparations only should be used. There will be situations, e.g. epilepsy, where it will be safer for the patient to be on her anticonvulsant drugs than to have a *grand mal* fit while crossing a busy main road. The balance of risk needs to be discussed with the patient, and documented in her records.

Maternity benefits

Information on a woman's eligibility for maternity benefits — which include Statutory Maternity Pay (SMP), Maternity Allowance, Sickness Benefit, and Additional Housing Benefit, Income Support and Family Credit — can be obtained from the antenatal clinic staff or the clinic's medical social worker.

Care plan for labour

In many hospitals women are invited to fill out a 'birthplan' for the conduct of their labour. This will cover all aspects of treatment a woman may receive when admitted in labour, to include the need for enema and perineal shave, mobility in labour, partner's presence at all times, early artificial rupturing of the membranes, electronic fetal heart rate monitoring, analgesia, position at delivery, the need for episiotomy, the timing of cord clamping, putting the baby to the breast, and keeping the baby in the delivery room. Sometimes a woman's wishes may initially be irritating to the medical team, but it is after all *her* baby and she should have some say as to what will be happening to her in labour. The 'birthplan' has the major advantage of involving the woman in her own management of labour. It does much to remove the criticism that she is regarded simply as a 'number' who has to comply with a rigid delivery policy. Most of the requests are reasonable, others will require discussion and compromise. There should never be a need for confrontation.

Subsequent antenatal visits

When a pregnancy is uncomplicated and there is no significant past medical or obstetric history that may indicate a need for particular investigations or more intensive antenatal monitoring, the normal fequency of antenatal checks is as follows:

Every 4 weeks until 28 weeks, then

Every 2 weeks until 36 weeks, then

Weekly until delivery.

In large maternity units, it would be impractical to carry out all these checks in the consultant unit antenatal clinic. Shared care with the GP and the community midwife is usual. There are advantages all round from this system of care. The GP continues to play a role in the care of the patient, who in turn usually finds it more convenient to attend the local surgery. The size of the consultant unit clinic is reduced, allowing time for more complex obstetric problems. The plan for shared care will vary between hospitals and indeed between different consultants in the same hospital. (See Table 2.1.)

When problems arise, consultant unit assessment will take the place of the GP assessment.

At every antenatal visit, whether at the consultant unit or GP clinic, the following details must be recorded:

- weight
- urinalysis
- blood pressure
- assessment of oedema
- abdominal examination.

Table 2.1 Plan for shared antenatal care

Place of antenatal appointment	Time
Initial GP assessment and referral	
Consultant unit booking appt.	8–12 weeks
〃 〃 reassessment	16 weeks
GP	20, 24 weeks
Consultant unit	28 weeks
GP	30, 32, 34 weeks
Consultant unit	36 weeks
GP	37, 38, 39 weeks
Consultant unit	40 weeks
〃 〃	41 weeks (? induction at 42 weeks)

It is usual for the woman to carry a Co-operation Card on which the findings at both the consultant and GP antenatal clinics are recorded.

Additional routine blood tests

- full blood count at   28 weeks & 36 weeks
- if rhesus-negative, for a   28 weeks & 36 weeks
  rhesus antibody screen at

Prophylactic iron/folic acid therapy

It has been traditional to give pregnant women prophylactic ferrous iron and folic acid during pregnancy. Although this has undoubtedly reduced the incidence of anaemia in the pregnant community, it is argued that in some women prophylaxis is unnecessary. If it is assumed that a good balanced diet alone is sufficient for *all* pregnant patients, then undoubtedly the incidence of anaemia in pregnancy will rise. **Prophylaxis is, therefore, either given to all women or to selected groups in the pregnant population.** The best predictor of the likelihood of developing an iron-deficiency anaemia is the serum ferritin level. (The cost of a single serum ferritin test is equal to the cost of standard cheap iron and folic acid therapy for 20 weeks.)

There is no doubt that severe anaemia increases the risks to both the woman and her fetus. For example, she will be less able to withstand the problems caused by severe haemorrhage if she is already anaemic. Intrauterine growth retardation and prematurity have also been linked to maternal anaemia.

If selection is to be carried out, the following groups of patients should receive prophylactic iron and folic acid:

(1) poor socio-economic groups;

(2) haemoglobin level of less than 11g/dl at booking;

(3) women with a past history of anaemia;

(4) multiple pregnancy;

(5) where there is evidence of blood loss e.g. recurrent antepartum bleeds, bleeding haemorrhoids.

If prophylactic iron and folic acid is to be given, there is little point in commencing this before the 20th week. If given earlier in the pregnancy, the iron preparation may exacerbate gastrointestinal symptoms which are common until about the 16th week, and discourage the patient from continuing with treatment for the duration of the pregnancy. It is essential to check on haemoglobin levels as outlined above. Patient compliance is not always the best it could be and it would be wrong to assume that anaemia cannot occur once treatment has commenced. The woman should be warned that she may experience either constipation or diarrhoea and that the motions will become black in colour. She should also be advised to keep the tablets out of reach of other small children in the family as the consequences of accidental consumption and overdosage in children can be fatal.

The third trimester

Once a pregnancy has passed the 24th week, the fetus in theory is viable. It would be foolhardy to assume that once this landmark has been reached, all will be well for the duration of the remainder of the pregnancy. Indeed, vigilance is increased as shown by the increased frequency of antenatal attendances.

The chief aims of antenatal care from the 26th week

(1) Detection of anaemia;

(2) detection of pregnancy-induced hypertension;

(3) assessment of uterine size and, after 34 weeks, the fetal lie, and presentation;

(4) detection of cephalo-pelvic disproportion (after 36 weeks);

(5) assessment of fetal well-being and antenatal fetal monitoring.

The clinical assessment of the pregnancy is based upon the findings at each attendance at the antenatal clinic, whether at a midwives' clinic, the GP surgery or the consultant unit.

Detection of anaemia

The routine full blood count taken at booking, 28 weeks and 36 weeks is the most commonly used means of detecting anaemia. The only *predictive* test that will indicate a likelihood of anaemia later in the pregnancy is a serum ferritin taken at booking.

Detection of pregnancy-induced hypertension

Routine measurement of the blood pressure at each antenatal visit is mandatory. In the very obese patient it is advisable to use a large cuff. After the 26th week, any blood pressure with a diastolic reading of 90 mm or more warrants admission of the woman for blood pressure assessment, *regardless of it returning to normal 10 minutes later*. Some hospitals are fortunate in having an antenatal assessment area where a woman may have her blood pressure assessed over a short period of time. If it should remain completely normal there would be no need for a full admission.

Assessment of uterine size, fetal lie, and presentation

Examination of the abdomen is carried out at each antenatal visit. Until 30 weeks, the chief purpose of abdominal palpation is to ensure that, clinically, the uterine size is compatible with the dates. A light touch with the flat of the examining hands will elicit much more information than a firm grip. Apart from hurting the woman, she will remember the experience and keep her abdominal muscles tense in readiness for the next manual assault on her uterus. While the fundal height on palpation, or measured in centimetres from the symphysis pubis, will give an indication of the period of gestation, this can be misleading. The true fundus is not always in the mid-line, and unless the whole of the abdomen is palpated, this fact can be missed (Fig. 2.2(a)). Sometimes the true fundus 'dips' away from the abdominal wall and, in error, it is assumed to be where it can be most easily palpated (Fig. 2.2(b)).

(a)

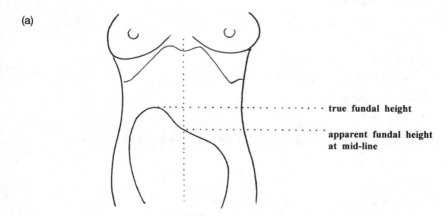

true fundal height

apparent fundal height at mid-line

Fig. 2.2   Illustrations (a) and (b) show how the true fundal height can be miscalculated if palpation is not carried out thoroughly.

(b)

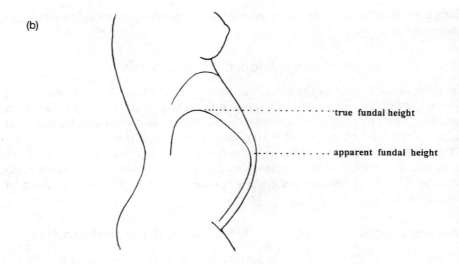

true fundal height

apparent fundal height

Fig. 2.2   (cont.)

Finally, in assessing the dates by palpation, the entire uterine size is taken into account. This will include the height and breadth of the uterus, the amount of liquor present, and the size of the fetus.

Having palpated the abdomen and determined the uterine size, the uterus will be found to be either compatible with dates,or large or small for dates.

The causes of date/size discrepancy in the third trimester

*Large for dates**

- wrong dates
- full bladder
- multiple pregnancy
- polyhydramnios (? fetal abnormality)
- uterine fibroids
- ovarian cyst.

Hydatidiform mole is excluded as it does not feature in the third trimester.

Small for dates

- wrong dates
- oligohydramnios (? fetal abnormality)
- placental insufficiency leading to intrauterine growth retardation.

There is little point in trying to determine the lie of the fetus or the presenting part until after the 30th week. The lie of the fetus is longitudinal, transverse, or oblique. After 32 weeks, the lie tends to become stable and remains longitudinal. If the lie is continually changing at successive examinations, it is described as being 'unstable'. The lie is often obvious on visual inspection of the abdomen. When the lie is longitudinal, the uterus appears to be elongated from the fundus towards the pelvic brim. When the lie is transverse, the uterus appears to be very broad and not very high in the abdomen. The actual lie is confirmed on examination by gently palpating downwards with both hands from the fundus of the uterus along its lateral contours to the pelvic brim.

The presenting part in a longitudinal lie is either cephalic or breech. (The term 'vertex' can only be used when the exact position of the head has been identified and other malpositions of the head have been excluded. This is usually only possible after vaginal, ultrasound or X-ray examination.) It is not always easy to be certain of the presenting part in a longitudinal lie. The patient may be very obese or the abdominal muscles very tense. If each fetal pole is held firmly between fingers and thumb, the fetal breech will eventually change its shape beneath the examining fingers with movement of the legs.

> If the head cannot be felt, it is either deeply engaged, under the ribs (breech presentation), or anencephalic.

The degree of engagement of the fetal head in the pelvis is noted at each abdominal examination. In the primigravida the head will generally commence to engage at 36 weeks, but in 10 per cent will only do so with the onset of labour. Among multiparous patients the head will usually only engage when labour commences. When the head is completely free with 5/5ths above the pelvic brim, it is mobile and can be ballotted gently from side to side between two hands. Once the head begins to enter the pelvis, its mobility disappears as it becomes 'fixed' in the pelvis. When engaged, the widest diameter of the head (biparietal diameter) is through the pelvic brim, and only 2/5ths of the head is felt abdominally. The only accurate way of assessing the degree of engagement of the head is by vaginal examination. The head has engaged when its lower pole is felt at the level of the ischial spines. (This is not always the case in labour, when caput can be at the level of the spines with the head not yet engaged.)

The position of the fetus antenatally (when not in labour) is determined by palpating the fetal back. Sometimes this can be found simply by visual inspection of the abdomen. If the fetal back is anterior, the flexed curve of the back gives the uterus a smooth convex curve from fundus to symphysis. In the occipito-posterior position, the fetal back is next to the maternal spine. This tends to result in a 'plateau' effect at the level of the umbilicus (the main value in correctly finding this sign is that it confirms your powers of observation and may impress an examiner during a clinical examination!). (See Fig. 2.3)

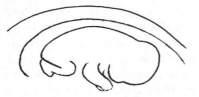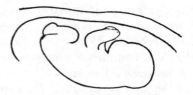

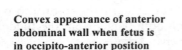

Convex appearance of anterior
abdominal wall when fetus is
in occipito-anterior position

"Plateau" appearance of anterior
abdominal wall when fetus is
in occipito-posterior position

Fig. 2.3 Illustrations to show how the appearance of the anterior abdominal wall
can give a clue to the lie of the fetus.

The commonest position is left occipito-lateral. The value of knowing the fetal
position antenatally is not great, but can be helpful in two ways. Firstly, it is
easier to auscultate the fetal heart with the Pinard stethoscope through the fetal
back. Secondly, it can be of value to know that the fetus is in an occipito-
posterior position. This is the commonest cause of a high head at term in a
primigravida, and may have implications for labour which tends to be longer
when there is this common malposition of the head.

Detection of cephalo-pelvic disproportion

Every primigravida is obviously an unknown quantity when it comes to actual
labour. Unless the head is high at term or the patient is of very short stature (less
than 150 cm), there is a regrettable tendency to assume that the pelvis will be
adequate and that if assessment is required it can always be left until she goes
into labour. Clinical assessment of the pelvis should be carried out in every
primigravida at 36–38 weeks. By this stage of pregnancy the fetal head is entering
the pelvic brim in the majority of primigravid patients. An engaged head gives
clear proof that there is no cephalo-pelvic disproportion at the pelvic brim.

> The best pelvimeter of the pelvic inlet is the fetal head.

When carrying out any vaginal examination after 36 weeks, a sterile glove as
opposed to a clean glove should always be used because of the greater likelihood
of labour occuring at this time. Chlorhexidine cream should be used as the
lubricant. The station of the fetal head is determined and cervical dilatation is
assessed.

At pelvic assessment the following questions must be answered:

1. Can the sacral promontory be felt?
2. If not already engaged, will the head enter the pelvis?
3. Is there a good concave sacral curve, is it flat or even convex?
4. Are the pelvic side walls convergent?
5. Are the ischial spines prominent?
6. Is the sub-pubic angle obtuse or acute?
7. Can the clenched fist be accommodated between the ischial tuberosities?

If there is any suggestion of cephalo-pelvic disproprtion at the pelvic brim, then further pelvimetry is required. Erect lateral pelvimetry by X-ray is becoming superseded by CAT scan pelvimetry when this is available.

Antenatal fetal monitoring

It is all too easy to relax one's vigilance once the pregnancy has safely reached viability. But sadly, Mother Nature is not always a very good midwife!

> The only safe policy in the last trimester of pregnancy is to actively look for problems rather than to await them.

There is no single test which will give absolute reassurance that all is well. Monitoring fetal well-being will be based upon clinical assessment and, in addition, may include:

- ultrasound assessment
- fetal kick chart
- antenatal cardiotocography
- biochemical screening (serial oestriol and human placental lactogen estimations).

Ultrasound assessment

Ultrasonography in the third trimester is not particularly helpful for dating purposes. The range for error can be as great as 2 weeks an either side of the actual date. Dating a pregnancy is best performed between 16 and 22 weeks. There are, however, two major benefits to be gained from ultrasonography in the third trimester. The first is the assessment of fetal growth, and the second, the accurate localization of the placental site.

Serial ultrasound measurements give valuable information regarding fetal growth. The most helpful measurements will be the biparietal diameter, abdominal circumference, and femur length. When placental insufficiency develops late in the pregnancy, glycogen stores in the fetal liver become depleted. This leads to a reduction in the growth rate of the liver and is the cause of slowing of the normal increase in abdominal circumference. Head growth is not immediately affected. As a result, intrauterine growth retardation due to placental insufficiency is asymmetrical or 'head sparing'. A single scan in itself will not be as helpful as serial scans carried out on a weekly or fortnightly basis.

Oligohydramnios is commonly found when there is placental insufficiency and contributes to the 'small-for-dates' uterus. Ultrasonography may detect this significant sign before it becomes clinically apparent.

Placental localization is dealt with in the section on antepartum haemorrhage.

Fetal kick chart

The purpose of the kick chart is for the woman herself to keep a daily eye on her baby's well-being, instead of only relying upon the check-ups made at her regular antenatal visits. From 28 weeks she is asked to record the time each day that she feels ten fetal movements. If she does not feel ten separate movements within the allotted 12 hours each day, she is instructed to ring the hospital concerned *that evening*. Cardiotocography (CTG) is then carried out. An abnormal CTG indicates the need for further review and sometimes delivery. Patient compliance depends on the clarity of explanation of the chart and the degree of enthusiasm and interest shown by the giver of the chart. It is very important that the woman understands that she is *never* wasting hospital time by having a CTG performed. She must not be tempted to put off contacting the hospital until the following day, even if she is seeing her midwife, GP, or consultant the next day. (See Fig. 2.4.)

The majority of women are very pleased to be involved in their own antenatal care. It is only a small minority of women who feel that they do not wish or have not got the time to count movements. Normal fetal movements indicate that there is unlikely to be a significant degree of fetal hypoxia *at that time*. Reduced

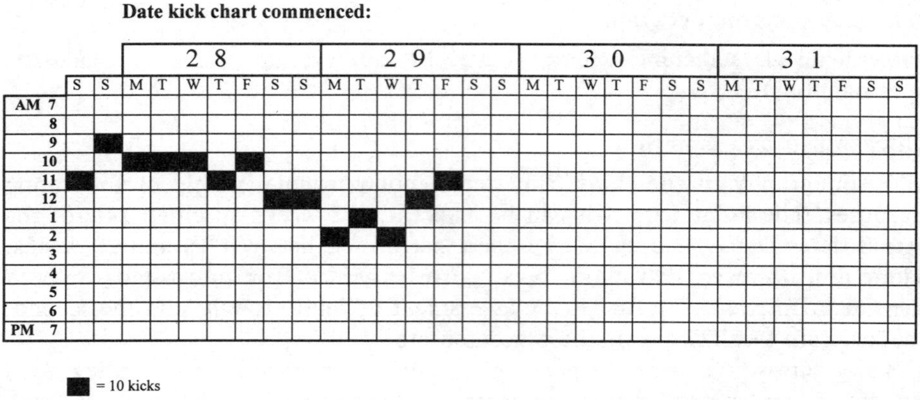

Date kick chart commenced:

	S	S	M	T	W	T	F	S	S	M	T	W	T	F	S	S	M	T	W	T	F	S	S	M	T	W	T	F	S	S
	\multicolumn{9}{c|}{2 8}									\multicolumn{7}{c|}{2 9}							\multicolumn{7}{c|}{3 0}							\multicolumn{7}{c|}{3 1}						
AM 7																														
8																														
9	■																													
10			■	■	■	■	■																							
11	■						■																							
12								■	■					■	■															
1													■																	
2										■	■																			
3																														
4																														
5																														
6																														
PM 7																														

■ = 10 kicks

Fig. 2.4 Example of kick chart.

fetal movements in themselves do not mean that there is a problem but do imply that reassurance must be sought by CTG.

Kick charts have been proven to save babies' lives. USE THEM!

Antenatal cardiotocography (CTG)

Cardiotocography gives valuable information on fetal well-being at the time that the recording is being made. This is the great advantage that CTG offers over biochemical tests. The results of biochemical investigations usually arrive 12–24 hours after the samples were collected and a single test result does not by itself give a useful indicator of fetal health.

There are a number of clinical situations when an antenatal CTG is carried out:

(1) on a regular out-patient basis, twice weekly as a routine form of monitoring;
(2) as a result of reduced fetal movements having been detected by the patient keeping a kick chart;
(3) as a daily assessment of in-patients where there is concern for fetal well-being.

The antenatal CTG is a 'non-stress test' of the fetus in that it records changes in the fetal heart rate in response to fetal movements and Braxton Hicks contractions. The 'cardiograph' is obtained by placing an external ultrasound transducer coated with coupling gel against the abdominal wall of the woman at the approximate level of the fetal heart. The 'tocograph' transducer which picks up uterine contractions is placed at the fundus of the uterus. Both transducers are held in position with rubber belts. It is important to ensure that there is no loss of contact between the fetal heart transducer and the maternal abdomen. To achieve this, in some patients it may be necessary for a midwife to be in attendance for the duration of the recording to hold the transducer firmly in place. The woman marks each fetal movement either electronically or manually onto the tracing. To be of any diagnostic value, the equipment used must be reliable and be capable of giving a good quality tracing. A poor quality machine is going to give an uninterpretable tracing and will only succeed in causing the woman unnecessary anxiety.

Each recording should last for at least 20 minutes, as there are normally frequent periods of fetal sleep when fetal heart rate variability and movement are both reduced. Too short a tracing that did not show the change back to normal fetal activity might otherwise be misinterpreted as showing hypoxic changes.

The normal CTG (see Fig. 2.5) will show:

(1) a fetal heart rate of between 120 and 160 beats per minute;
(2) good variability of at least 15 beats per minute;

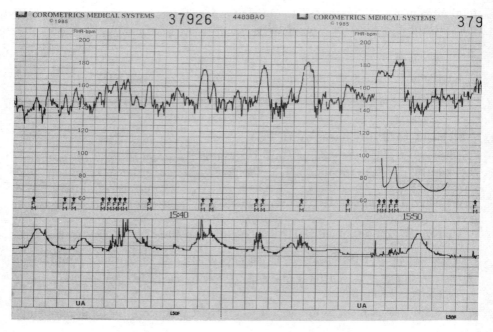

Fig. 2.5   CTG tracing showing normal fetal heart rate.

(3) normal accelerations of the fetal heart rate in response to both fetal movement and Braxton Hicks contractions;

(4) the presence of fetal movements.

If there is a very prolonged apparent 'sleep' pattern, the CTG should be continued for a further 20 minutes in order to give an opportunity for normal 'waking' activity to return (see Fig. 2.6). Sometimes 'waking' can be gently encouraged by abdominal palpation of the uterus.

> It must not be assumed that a tracing that shows a prolonged 'sleep' pattern for over 20 minutes is normal. SEEK ADVICE.

The abnormal CTG (see Fig. 2.7) may show the following features:

(1) a normal baseline fetal heart rate or a rate above 160 beats per minute,

(2) reduced or absent variability;

(3) no accelerations in fetal heart rate in response to fetal movement and Braxton Hicks contractions (non-reactive);

(4) decelerations in fetal heart rate.

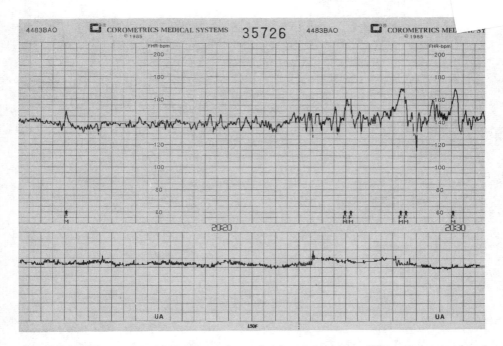

Fig. 2.6 CTG tracing showing prolonged 'sleep' pattern, followed by 'waking' activity.

Any deceleration of the fetal heart rate on an antenatal CTG must be regarded as being potentially ominous. SEEK ADVICE.

It must be remembered that if it is decided to induce labour as a result of a worrying and abnormal CTG, the fetus will be subjected to a 'stress' situation, once strong contractions become established. It may be considered to be safer to deliver a premature, growth-retarded fetus via the abdominal route.

Biochemical screening

Before the ready availability of antenatal cardiotocography and serial ultrasonography, obstetricians put considerable reliance upon biochemical screening tests as a means of monitoring fetal well-being. Because at best the results give retrospective information, their importance is declining.

Urinary oestriol measurements are made either from a 24-hour urine collection or as an oestriol/creatinine ratio from an early-morning urine collection. Plasma oestrial levels are preferred by some clinicians. As oestriol is the end product of

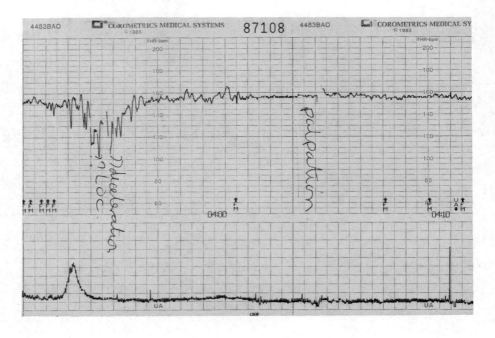

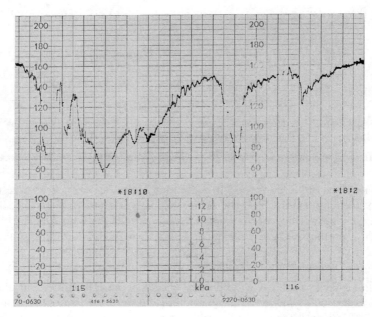

Fig. 2.7   (a) Moderately abnormal CTG tracing; (b) severely abnormal CTG.

fetal androgens which have been converted by a placental sulphatase enzyme, the oestriol level gives a guide to the normal function of the feto–placental unit. If the fetus is compromised by placental insufficiency, the oestriol level will fall. It should be noted that if fetal androgen output is minimal, as occurs in the anencephalic fetus or the rare condition of congenital adrenal hypoplasia, the corresponding oestriol levels are extremely low. Very occasionally there can be a deficiency in the placental sulphatase enzyme which will also be associated with very low oestriol levels.

A single low oestriol level is of little prognostic value, and indicates a need for further monitoring by means of serial oestriol estimations and cardiotocography in order to be able to give any indication of reduced fetal well-being.

Human Placental Lactogen (HPL) is a placental hormone which is produced in increasing quantities until term is reached. Maternal blood levels of HPL can be used as an indication of normal placental function. As with oestriol, a single result is not helpful and is always retrospective. A trend of static or falling HPL levels indicates a need for further monitoring.

The decision to deliver a baby, where there is cause for concern, is based upon a combination of the patient's history, clinical assessment, and the results of screening. Most obstetricians will have experienced the distressing and disconcerting situation of a sudden, unexplained intrauterine death, where a CTG only hours earlier had been normal. Similarly, stillbirths can occur when the oestriols, HPLs and kick chart have all been normal until the day of fetal death. Fortunately, this is an unusual occurrence.

Prenatal diagnosis

Fetal abnormalities are extremely common, but the vast majority will abort spontaneously in the first trimester. The remainder will be delivered as babies with an inherited disorder or congenital malformation. As most congenital abnormalities are incurable, many of these babies will not survive beyond infancy. Of those that do, the majority will require many years of medical care and be a cause of great distress to the parents. Most couples, once fully informed and counselled, will elect to prevent the birth of an abnormal baby by means of termination of that pregnancy.

Two to three per cent of couples have a high risk in every pregnancy of having children with an inherited disorder.

One to two per cent of babies are born with a congenital abnormality, the majority to young and healthy women with no identifiable risk factors.

The aims of prenatal diagnosis are clear:

(1) to ensure that couples at risk of having an abnormal baby can come to an informed decision as to their options;

(2) to allow 'at risk' couples to have the confidence to embark upon a pregnancy in the knowledge that a termination of pregnancy will be available in the event of a major abnormality being detected;

(3) to reassure any woman who would wish to be screened, that her pregnancy has no detectable abnormality, and so greatly alleviate worry and distress.

The diagnosis of fetal abnormality cannot be made before pregnancy. As most of these babies are born to healthy women under the age of 35 years, their detection can only be improved upon by carrying out 'blanket screening' on *all* pregnant women who wish to be screened.

Maternal serum alpha-fetoprotein screening (AFP)

Maternal serum AFP screening *alone* will detect the majority of open neural tube defects, i.e. 90 per cent of anencephalic fetuses and 80 per cent of spina bifida fetuses. This is not as high a failure rate as it seems, bearing in mind that the national incidence of neural tube defects ranges between 3 and 8 per 1000 births.

AFP screening for neural tube defects should *not* be carried out as a blanket screening on every woman without informing her first and discussing any queries that may arise. Considerable alarm can otherwise be caused simply by mentioning that a blood test to exclude spina bifida is performed routinely on every patient. The aim of the test should be explained, giving her the chance to opt out if that is her wish. At the time of counselling her about AFP screening, she should be made aware of what the next steps would be in the event of a raised 'screen-positive' result. If a termination of pregnancy would not be considered under any circumstances, there may at first seem to be no point in carrying out the test. However, couples in this situation will often appreciate knowing if there is an abnormality so that they and other members of the family will have the opportunity of accustoming themselves to the problem before delivery.

There is no value in carrying out this test on a known multiple pregnancy as the level is going to be raised in any case and therefore meaningless. If a woman has had a threat to miscarry earlier in the preqnancy, she should be warned that her AFP level may be raised because of the feto-maternal transfusion of blood that frequently occurs at such an event. This advice could save her some anxious moments, even though further screening will still be necessary.

Ideally, the AFP test is carried out at 15–16 weeks, allowing ample time for further screening if required. While a 'screen-negative' result will have exluded the majority of open neural tube defects, it is important that the woman appreciates that a normal AFP level does not guarantee a normal baby. A 'screen-positive' result will be above the 95th centile. (See Fig. 2.8.)

When a raised AFP level is found, the woman must be asked to return to the clinic. To allay her very understandable fears she should be told that **the majority of patients with a raised AFP level will have a normal pregnancy**, the raised result being due to wrong dates, multiple pregnancy, threatened miscarriage earlier in the pregnancy, and for no detectable reason in some patients. The AFP test is repeated and a scan (if not already performed) is carried out to confirm dates and exclude a multiple pregnancy. If the second result is also elevated, the next

Graph for the interpretation of AFP results in Pregnancy

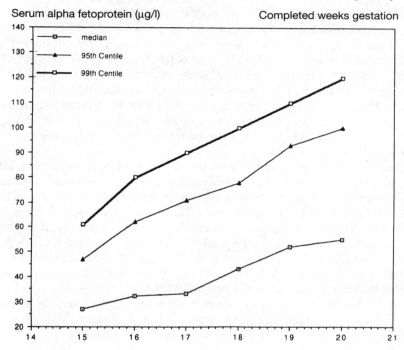

Fig. 2.8 Graph for the interpretation AFP results in pregnancy.

step will vary in different units, the choice being between detailed ultrasonography, amniocentesis, or both.

> Ten per cent of patients with a raised AFP have a fetal abnormality.

Fetal abnormalities will include:

- open neural tube defects:, spina bifida, anencephaly
- exomphalos
- gut atresias
- ectopia vesicae
- fetal nephrotic syndrome.

Detailed ultrasonography

Between 18 and 22 weeks nearly all major abnormalities can be detected with detailed ultrasonography. As 90 per cent of such abnormalities occur in the pregnancies of young healthy women who are not generally considered to be at risk, the only way to detect more is to offer detailed ultrasonography to all women. Some obstetricians feel that because of the distress caused by AFP screening, this test should be abandoned for a routine detailed ultrasound on all patients. There are, however, implications of the cost of medical and ultrasound staff and equipment and, perhaps most of all, of medical time. This is particularly relevant in a large unit. It must be remembered that it takes 15 minutes to carry out a detailed scan.

A detailed ultrasound scan at 18 weeks should be able to detect virtually all neural tube defects. A skilled ultrasonographer can even suspect an undetectable spina bifida from changes in the lemon-shape of the fetal head and banana-shape of the cerebellum. There is rarely any difficulty in establishing a diagnosis of anencephaly. If the detailed scan is completely normal, especially in the woman with only a marginally raised serum AFP, it is usually decided that no further screening is required. In a twin pregnancy, serum AFP screening cannot be used to detect a neural tube defect. However, a detailed scan at 18 weeks can give considerable reassurance as to the normality of both fetuses.

At 18–22 weeks the normality of other structures apart from the brain and spine can also be determined. The heart, kidneys, bladder, abdominal wall, diaphragm, and limbs can be clearly screened.

Amniocentesis

The aim of amniocentesis is to obtain a sample of amniotic fluid for further study. In many units this is still only being performed at 16 weeks. However, amniocentesis can be safely undertaken at 13–14 weeks. *Early amniocentesis* at 10 weeks is now being evaluated, the problems being that the cell harvest is low and the failure rate high. When counselling a woman for amniocentesis, it is important to ensure that she is aware of the small risk of spontaneous abortion as a direct result of the test. This occurs in approximately 0.75–1 per cent of cases and can occur within 4 weeks of the amniocentesis. Furthermore, she must realize that if she did abort, it would be a normal fetus that would be lost. There is also an increased incidence of premature labour and abruptio placentae. [**It is very much in the interests of the doctor that any advice given to the patient is documented and dated in her case notes.**]

The amniocentesis is carried out after ultrasound localization of the placenta and ideally under ultrasound control, so that the most suitable liquor pool is used for sampling. The patient must have an empty bladder. It does not help you or the patient to send urine and not liquor to the laboratory!

Procedure: The skin is cleaned. A bleb of local anaesthetic is raised in the skin with a fine needle. A further 5 ml of 1% lignocaine is injected through the abdominal

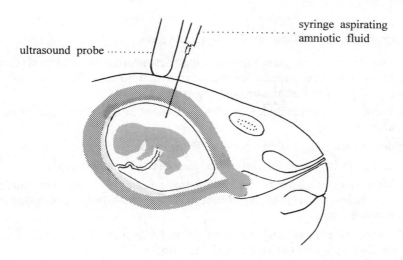

ultrasound probe

syringe aspirating
amniotic fluid

Fig. 2.9 Amniocentesis.

wall and uterine wall. Sometimes the No. 1 needle used for administering the lignocaine will penetrate the amnion and liquor is withdrawn with ease. Usually this is not the case, especially in the woman with a thicker abdominal wall. A 22 gauge spinal needle is inserted into the amniotic cavity. It is always worth while to discard the first ml of liquor so as to avoid contamination with maternal cells if a karyotyping of the fetus is also being quested. (See Fig. 2.9.)

After the amniocentesis has been performed, the patient should rest for half an hour before gently going home. (In the rhesus-negative, unsensitized patient, unless the father is also rhesus-negative, 125 μg of anti-D immunoglobulin is administered routinely within 72 hours of the test.)

If the liquor AFP is more than three times the median for the gestation, then there is a very high likelihood of an abnormality. The diagnostic accuracy can be increased by measuring the liquor acetyl cholinesterase which is a normal constituent of fetal cerebrospinal fluid. In an open neural tube defect, CSF mixes with the amniotic fluid.

If an amniocentesis is being performed, it would be sensible to take advantage of the test and also send liquor for karyotyping.

There are also many inheritable biochemical and metabolic disorders which may be specifically screened for by amniocentesis. The list of detectable conditions is constantly growing, and the advice of a geneticist or neonatologist should be sought if there is a significant family history.

Summary of the indications for amniocentsesis

(1) The detection of raised liquor alpha-fetoprotein in suspected cases of neural tube defect. Further confirmation may be obtained by measuring the liquor acetyl cholinesterase;

(2) karyotyping to exclude Down's syndrome and other chromosomal abnormalities;

(3) determining fetal sex in sex-linked disorders;

(4) detection of numerous inherited disorders of metabolism;

(5) assessment of severity of rhesus iso-immunization by determining the optical density of the liquor (this has now been superseded by cordocentesis);

(6) determining fetal lung maturity prior to delivery by measuring the lecithin/sphyngomyelin ratio (L/S ratio).

Karyotyping

From the age of 35 years, the subject of karyotyping to exclude Down's syndrome should at least be discussed with every antenatal patient. If the woman would not wish for any action to be taken in the event of an abnormal karyotype, then that would be the end of the matter and her wishes should be documented on the notes. In order to be able to give balanced counselling and compare the risks of the procedure with the likelihood of detecting a problem, it is of course essential to know the approximate incidence of Down's syndrome for any particular age group.

The approximate incidence of Down's syndrome in relation to increasing maternal age

At 30 years	1 in 1000
35 years	1 in 380
36 years	1 in 300
37 years	1 in 240
38 years	1 in 180
39 years	1 in 140
40 years	1 in 100
42 years	1 in 80
44 years	1 in 40
46 years	1 in 20

It is very important that the risk of Down's syndrome is kept in perspective. It can be seen from the above table that, even at the age of 46, the odds are very much in favour of a normal karyotype.

The chief indications for karyotyping the fetus

(1) increasing maternal age;

(2) a previous pregnancy affected with Down's syndrome or other chromosomal abnormality;

(3) to determine the fetal sex in sex-linked disorder, e.g. haemophilia, Duchenne's muscular dystrophy, where there is a 50 per cent risk of a male fetus being affected;

(4) peace of mind.

In very skilled hands, amniocentesis can be carried out on a twin pregnancy using careful ultrasound guidance. The miscarriage rate will be increased, since if one twin were to miscarry, the other would be lost as well. The patient must also be aware of the problems that could arise if, say, one twin was found to have an abnormal karyotype and the other was normal. It is now possible to consider the selective fetocide of the affected twin, rather than put the couple through the awful dilemma of whether or not to terminate the entire pregnancy, including the normal twin. However, this is fraught with ethical and legal problems.

Occasionally a woman in her twenties will be terrified at even the remotest chance of Down's syndrome affecting her baby. In such cases quoting statistics and 'the odds' are meaningless. As long as she is clearly aware of the risks, karyotyping is reasonable so as to allow her to enjoy her pregnancy without being in a state of terror for the remaining months.

Sometimes a woman will request that a karyotype is carried out simply because she wishes to know the sex of the baby. The usual reason for this is that she only has daughters and is desperate to have a son, or vice versa. However, the risks of the test do not justify the indication. Detailed scanning by a skilled ultrasonographer should be able to sex the baby with a fair degree of accuracy—but, a word of caution. Ultrasound sexing is not foolproof and the patient *must* be advised of this. Medico–legal problems have arisen from incorrect ultrasound sexing. It may become apparent that there are major family pressures on her, where both her husband and in-laws are blaming her for not providing a son and grandson. Should this be the case, it is very worth while to first see the couple and explain not some simple genetics to them, pointing out that whether or not she has a son is up to him! Very occasionally obstetricians are asked if they will determine the sex of the baby and terminate the pregnancy if the baby should prove to be 'yet another girl'. To carry out this request would be a criminal offence. Even if the woman would not wish to go as far as termination, she would have the months ahead to resent a baby of the 'wrong' sex.

The two major techniques for obtaining material in order to karyotype a fetus are **chorion villus sampling (CVS)** and **amniocentesis.**

(The technique of **coelocentesis** is currently being evaluated. Coelomic fluid in the extra-embryonic coelomic cavity surrounds the amniotic sac and can be aspirated as early as 6–10 weeks. The advantage of coelocentesis over amniocentesis is that the amnion is not punctured, which reduces the risk of fetal trauma. The advantage over CVS is that the placenta is not disturbed. The risks have still to be assessed.)

Chorion villus sampling (CVS)

The option of CVS is only available to those women who present early enough in the pregnancy, the test being performed at 10 weeks. If the woman herself has only realized that she was pregnant after this date, or if the GP is unaware of the investigation options and refers the patient for booking at 12 weeks, then amniocentesis will be the only option. The big advantage of CVS is that a diagnosis is reached before the 12th week, considerably reducing the stress that will affect most couples. If a termination of pregnancy is required, this can still be performed under general anaesthesia.

Procedure: Under ultrasound control, a fine needle is passed either via the cervix or transabdominally (depending upon placental site) and aspirates a small biopsy of chorionic villi; 20–50 mg of tissue is required for diagnostic purposes. (See Fig. 2.10.)

Advantages and disadvantages of CVS versus amniocentesis

CVS	Amniocentesis
• performed after 10 weeks	• performed at 10–16 weeks
• result within 72 hours	• result within 4 weeks
• karyotype & DNA analysis	• karyotype & liquor for AFP & DNA analysis
• up to 2 per cent miscarriage risk	• up to 1 per cent miscarriage risk
• up to 1 per cent limb deformity risk if performed before 10 weeks	
• early termination if required	• late termination if required.

Although the abortion rate is higher after CVS, it is difficult to determine whether this is entirely due to the test itself, as the spontaneous abortion rate itself is highest during the first trimester. Many women will prefer to have the diagnosis made earlier rather than have to face a late prostaglandin termination

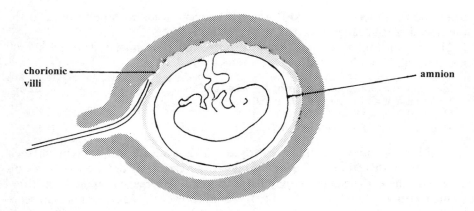

chorionic
villi

amnion

Fig. 2.10   Chorion villus sampling.

of pregnancy should this be required. On the other hand, if there has been a past history of miscarriages or if the pregnancy has been at all unstable, with threats to miscarry, then amniocentesis with its lower miscarriage risk may be the preferred procedure. It is important that the woman understands that if she does miscarry after the test has been performed, the overwhelming odds are that the aborted pregnancy was normal.

Pregnant women who are 35 years of age and over, account for only some 6 per cent of the total pregnant population. Yet this small group produces 20 per cent of the Down's syndrome babies. The 94 per cent of younger women below the age of 35 produce the remaining 80 per cent of cases. The only way to pick up more cases of Down's syndrome will be to carry out more karyotyping and to include younger patients in the screening programme. Yet it is generally accepted that amniocentesis should only be carried out when the risk of finding an abnormality is greater than the risk of fetal loss, i.e. when the abnormality risk is greater than 1 in 200. The problem, therefore, is to find the at-risk patients in the younger age group.

Biochemical screening for risk of Down's syndrome

Three biochemical markers have been found to be associated with a Down's syndrome fetus:

- maternal serum AFP level is significantly lowered
- free beta-hCG is raised
- unconjugated oestriol (uE_3) is lowered

Some centres are using these markers as a 'triple test' — in addition to maternal age — to detect the 'screen-positive' patients, where the risk of having a Down's syndrome pregnancy is assessed as being 1 in 200 or more. The blood sample that is used for the current AFP test provides the means to test for hCG and

uE_3. The sensitivity of the AFP assay, however, needs to be improved at the lower end of the range.

The proportion of Down's syndrome-affected pregnancies detected should increase significantly:

Maternal age alone, all women of 35 years and over	20%
Maternal age and maternal serum AFP	37%
Maternal age, AFP and hCG	57%
Maternal age, AFP, hCG ind uE_3	63%

Health authorities will find the 'triple test' is a cost-effective item on their budget if the detection of Down's babies is increased. In order to achieve this objective, the entire antenatal population should be screened, apart from those women who would wish to opt out. It would, however, make economical sense to drop the oestriol estimation as this adds little to the pick-up rate. For those patients with a risk of between 1 in 200 and 1 in 400, the introduction of a neutrophil alkaline phosphatase test may be considered as a secondary screening. Although this test is expensive, a raised result would dramatically increase the pick-up rate.

There will be two interesting results of such screening. Firstly, some women in the older age group who traditionally would have wanted, and been offered, karyotyping, will be found to be 'screen-negative' and not wish to have an amniocentesis. Secondly, the number of amniocenteses in the younger age group will increase, dramatically increasing the pressure on clinical genetic services. There will also be an increase in the number of abortions of normal pregnancies resulting from the hunt for more Down's syndrome pregnancies.

> Remember that both the 'double' and 'triple test' are specific for trisomy 21 (Down's syndrome) and will NOT detect the other trisomies.

Karyotyping will detect other chromosomal problems such as Turner's syndrome (45XO), Klinefelter's syndrome (47XXY) and XYY syndrome. These will also increase with maternal age. There will be a need for expert genetic counselling in the event of such conditions being found.

> For women who are over the age of 40, amniocentesis rather than blood screening should be advised.

If a termination of pregnancy is decided upon as a result of the findings of screening, it is obvious that this is going to be associated with considerable anguish and distress for the couple. If a second trimester termination is required with the use of prostaglandins, the ideal environment will be the labour ward where there are epidural facilities. Many couples express a wish to see and handle the baby and, indeed, this should be encouraged. If the couple should choose not to see the baby, then photography is important in the event of the couple requesting a picture at a later date (see section on perinatal death, p. 239).

Fetoscopy

This is a technique performed under ultrasound control, which permits visual inspection of the baby by means of a fine telescope which is passed into the amniotic cavity via the abdominal wall. Fetal blood sampling from the insertion of the cord can then be carried out. The spontaneous abortion rate following this specialized procedure is between 3 and 7 per cent.

Cordocentesis

With the advances in ultrasound, it is no longer necessary to carry out fetal blood sampling via a fetoscope. In skilled hands, a fine needle is passed through the abdominal wall, and a blood sample taken directly from the cord. If the placenta is anterior, the operator can obtain the blood sample by passing the needle through the placenta to the 'root' of the cord at its insertion (Fig. 2.11). As the needle used is much finer than the fetoscope, the pregnancy loss following cordocentesis is reduced.

Indications for cordocentesis

(1) detection of fetal haemoglobinopathies such as sickle-cell disease and thalassaemia where both parents are carriers of the trait;

(2) detection of sex-linked disorders once a male fetus has been found at amniocentesis or CVS in a known carrier, e.g, haemophilia;

(3) to determine the fetal blood group;

(4) to determine the severity of rhesus iso-immunization and as an improved method of intrauterine transfusion in a very severely affected baby;

(5) to rapidly karyotype the fetus;

The scope of prenatal diagnosis is increasing rapidly. For the screening of the pregnant population to increase in the future, the development of more screening centres is vital. Obstetricians specializing in fetal medicine and clinical geneticists backed up by laboratory diagnostic specialists, are now recognized as an essential part of modern obstetrics.

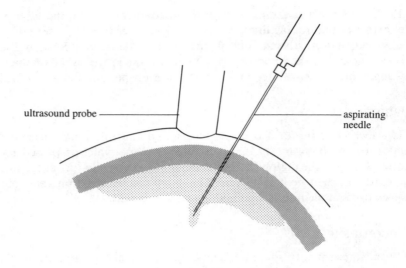

ultrasound probe ————————————————— aspirating
needle

Fig. 2.11   Cordocentesis when placenta is anterior.

Infection screening

The effects on the fetus of maternal infection depend directly upon the infecting organism and its virulence. Severe major infections associated with a high pyrexia will lead to early abortion or intrauterine death. Less severe infections will rarely cause problems, with the exception of toxoplasmosis, rubella, and cytomegalovirus. These three, with the addition of herpes simplex, form the so-called TORCH infections. They will be considered here among other causes of infection that are either screened for routinely or may require screening for in certain circumstances.

Rubella

The risks to the fetus of rubella infection in the early weeks of pregnancy are well documented. It is not until well into the second trimester that the fetus's own immune system becomes competent to protect itself. The majority of pregnant women in the UK are immune to rubella, whether or not they have had any history of having had this mild infection. Fifteen per cent of women are found to have no rubella immunity. However, many pregnant women will not know whether they are immune to rubella. A history of having had the illness or even the vaccination is not sufficient as other viral infections can mimic rubella and 5 per cent of the vaccinations fail to give immunity.

At the booking appointment blood is routinely taken to screen for rubella immunity, unless it is already known from a previous recent test that the woman is immune. If she is not immune, the notes should be clearly documented so that vaccination can be given postnatally. If a non-immune patient comes into contact with rubella or develops any symptoms suggestive of the condition, blood should be taken as soon as possible for re-testing. A rapid rise in rubella antibodies in two consecutive tests taken 2 weeks apart will confirm the diagnosis. The risk of a major congenital malformation is 50 per cent during the first 6 weeks, falling to 30 per cent by 12 weeks. Therapeutic termination of pregnancy is usually offered to all women who are proven to have contracted rubella during the first trimester.

Hepatitis B

Hepatitis B antigen (Australia antigen) is now screened for routinely by regional blood transfusion centres when blood-grouping is performed. Antenatal clinics are informed of any positive result. In the event of there not being a routine screening service, screening should be carried out on women who are known drug abusers, who have had tattoos, or who have come from areas of the world where hepatitis B is relatively common. The main risk antenatally is to the attendant medical, nursing, and laboratory staff who will come into contact with blood, urine, faeces and amniotic fluid. (For this reason, medical and ancilliary staff are strongly recommended to seek vaccination against hepatitis B.)

There does not appear to be a significant risk to the patient or fetus antenatally, but the newborn baby can become infected as a result of swallowing infected liquor or blood during labour. These patients require barrier nursing when admitted.

Toxoplasmosis

Public awareness is increasing with regard to this protozoal infection. The host of this parasite is the domestic cat. Pregnant women should avoid the handling of cat faeces and cat litter trays. Infection can also be contracted from handling uncooked meat that has been contaminated by cat faeces. Simple hygiene is of obvious importance. Toxoplasmosis infections in the human are largely asymptomatic. They are, however, a cause of spontaneous and recurrent abortion, stillbirth, and major neurological problems in the baby. It is possible to screen women for this infection, but its relatively low incidence in the UK would make routine screening on all pregnant women an expensive programme to undertake. It may be worth while to consider the screening of all pregnant women who are cat owners. If a positive screening test is obtained in early pregnancy it raises the question of either antibiotic therapy or possibly termination of pregnancy.

Cytomegalovirus (CMV)

This virus is relatively common, affecting up to 4 per cent of pregnant women. The main means of transmission is by saliva, usually from children to the adult. The infection is asymptomatic, but can cause recurrent abortion, intrauterine death, intrauterine growth retardation, mental retardation, cerebral palsy, and microcephaly. Up to 20 per cent of the babies will have a congenital anomaly resulting from this infection. The baby will become infected either by the virus crossing the placenta, or from contact with the cervix at delivery, or even breast feeding. The condition can be detected by a rising antibody titre, but antenatal screening does not give any guidance as to whether or not the fetus is affected. Furthermore, some women will only become infected late in the pregnancy. Prevention of this condition is impossible until a vaccine is developed.

Herpes simplex

The herpes simplex type II virus is transmitted by intercourse and commonly infects the lower genital tract. The presence of painful shallow ulcers over the vulva, vagina, or cervix should suggest the diagnosis. Prompt referral to a genito–urinary clinic is indicated so that appropriate culture of the virus can be carried out. If positive, antiviral therapy is required. A new primary infection occuring in pregnancy puts the baby at greater risk than a recurrent infection.

The major time of risk for the baby is during vaginal delivery, when it may come into prolonged contact with actively infected tissues. If there is active herpes prior to labour, confirmed on culture, it is then undoubtedly safer to deliver the baby electively by Caesarean section.

Acquired Immune Deficiency Syndrome (AIDS)

The general public are familiar with the potential problems of contracting AIDS as a result of exposure to the human immunovirus (HIV). There is no policy of screening all pregnant women and it is generally accepted that screening should not be carried out except with the consent of the individual concerned. Many antenatal clinics have leaflets which are presented to women at booking, where at-risk groups are highlighted and patients in such groups are asked to put themselves forwards for HIV screening.

> It must be remembered that there will be pregnant *unscreened* women who have HIV antibodies and that when screening is being carried out, it is in the interests of the woman herself and not in the interests of the staff attending her.

The following groups of patients should be considered for screening:

(1) sexual contacts of homosexual and bisexual men;
(2) drug abusers who inject drugs or whose sexual contact injects drugs;
(3) women who themselves or whose sexual contacts have lived in areas where AIDS is endemic, such as sub-Sahara, Central, and East Africa, and Haiti;
(4) sexual contacts of haemophiliac patients who have been treated with blood products;
(5) any patient who requests screening.

Pregnancy appears to convert HIV-positive patients into full AIDS and their babies have a significant risk of being born with the disease. Because of this risk, HIV-positive pregnant women are offered termination of pregnancy if they book early enough. If the offer of termination is refused by the woman after she has been fully counselled of the risks to herself and her baby, or if the diagnosis is only made late in pregnancy, she should have full hospital antenatal care carried out by one senior obstetrician. Specimens are handled as for hepatitis B carriers. Labour, delivery, and postnatal care are similarly dealt with as for hepatitis B carriers.

Special patient groups

Ethnic minorities

Many cities in the UK have large thriving immigrant populations. For many, especially among the Asian communities, English is a second language and there are undoubted problems of communication. However, not only have antenatal information books been translated into Hindi, Punjabi, Gujarati, Bengali, and Urdu, but some antenatal clinics are staffed by 'link workers' who can bridge the communication gap between clinic staff and patients. Ideally the link worker should herself belong to the ethnic minority involved but have been educated within the majority community. Hospital staff need to understand the different social environment, religious customs, and dietary regulations. The woman must understand the importance of antenatal care, adequate diet, the possible need for supplementary calcium and vitamin D, the benefits to which she is entitled, and how and where to seek help. The perinatal mortality rate among the Asian community is approximately double that of the Caucasian population. For this reason, it is advisable that the majority of Asian women should be delivered in the Consultant unit.

The main antenatal problems to be aware of include

- anaemia
- haemoglobinopathies
- TB
- tropical diseases (e.g. malaria)
- disproportion.

The woman herself is often small in stature and generally has smaller than average babies. With the improvement in diet and health, babies have tended to become larger with an increased incidence of disproportion.

Whether antenatally or in labour, communication is of the utmost importance. It is all too easy in a busy antenatal clinic to simply nod and smile at someone who does not understand a word that is being said to her. Similarly, when in labour, it must be remembered that from the point of view of many of these women, they are in a foreign country, do not understand what is being done to them and, very reasonably, are frightened.

The Afro-Caribbean population in general do not have the problem of a language barrier. For both clinical and medico–legal considerations, it should be routine to screen all such patients for sickle-cell disease.

The elderly primigravida

Primigravidae over the age of 35 years are regarded as being older than average to have their first baby. Some clinicians feel that this age should be brought down to include women over the age of 30 years. When discussing the potential problems of increased maternal age, it is important to be factual and not allow the woman to feel as if she is a dinosaur! When taking the history, it is significant to determine the reason for the 'late start' in having a family. This may be due to involuntary infertility or be voluntary because of a career. On the other hand, she may have only recently married and not had an earlier opportunity to become pregnant. A pregnancy that occurs after treatment for long-standing infertility has a high premium, as this may be the only pregnancy she will have. As a result, antenatal care will be more intensive, the consultant unit usually carrying out the bulk of the care. Additional antenatal fetal monitoring with serial ultrasonography is recommended.

The chief antenatal problems of the elderly primigravida will include:

- abortion
- pre-existing gynaecological problems such as fibroids
- karyotyping for Down's syndrome (depending on age)
- hypertensive disorders
- intrauterine growth retardation
- premature labour.

There should be ready recourse to admission should any significant antenatal problem arise.

For vaginal delivery to be contemplated, the pelvis must be beyond reproach, and the presentation of the fetus must be cephalic.

An elderly primigravida plus a complication is considered to be an indication for an elective Caesarean section.

Pregnancy should not be allowed to go much past term. Induction of labour is generally not a problem. As instrumental or operative delivery is a frequent occurence, the use of epidural anaesthesia from the onset of labour is strongly recommended. The fetus must be continuously monitored in labour and delivered by the speediest route should problems arise. Increased maternal age has been shown to increase the incidence of postpartum haemorhage. It is important that the woman understands the plan of management and is reassured by the close monitoring of both the fetus and her own progress in labour.

> There is no place for a trial of labour, vaginal breech delivery, or vaginal twin delivery in the elderly primigravida.

The grand multipara

The 'grand multip' is a woman having her fifth or subsequent baby. Most commonly she is of low socio-economic class and it is this that contributes to her antenatal problems. She is usually worn out by the demands of her large family, with pregnancies that have rapidly followed each other. She eats poorly, is often grossly obese, gets insufficient rest and sleep, and has poor dentition because she is too busy to look after herself and visit a dentist regularly. The minor antenatal ailments such as varicose veins and haemorrhoids can be particularly troublesome.

The grand multipara must be booked for delivery in the Consultant Unit. Her attendance at antenatal clinics will often be poor as she 'has not got the time'. Because her previous labours have usually been rapid, she assumes that having another baby is going to be like 'shelling peas' and therefore is not impressed by medical advice. She will often resist admission, unless it is to be delivered.

The combination of poor general health, her older age group, and a lax, overstretched uterus, produce the problems she may face antenatally and in labour.

Antenatal problems of the 'grand multip'

(1) **anaemia**;

(2) **poor general health** and malnutrition;

(3) **hypertensive disorders**;

(4) **abruptio placentae** associated with pregnancy-induced hypertension;

(5) **unstable lie** and associated malpresentations due to the lax uterus;

(6) risk of **cord prolapse** should spontaneous rupture of the membranes occur;

(7) **cephalo–pelvic disproportion** due to the tendency for babies to get larger in successive pregnancies and subluxation forwards of the sacrum on the sacroiliac joints, thereby reducing the antero-posterior diameter at the pelvic brim.

The main problems in labour are due to the ability of the 'grand multip's uterus to contract over-efficiently as it is highly sensitive to endogenous oxytocin.

> **If labour is to be induced in the grand multipara, oxytocics must NEVER be used.**

It is safer to think in terms of an elective Caesarean section in the grand multipara rather than to attempt to deliver a very large baby vaginally. There is no place for a trial of labour if cephalo–pelvic disproportion is suspected.

> **The problems in labour in the grand multipara**
>
> - precipitate labour (less than 4 hours)
> - uterine rupture caused by titanic contractions especially where there is unrecognized obstruction
> - postpartum haemorrhage, due to a prolonged uterine relaxation phase after the rapid delivery of the baby.

Premature labour with a breech presentation should be managed with an epidural anaesthetic if there is time to insert one. The grand multipara will not be able to resist pushing with contractions and can usually deliver the baby up to the neck through an incompletely dilated cervix. A cervix clamped around the neck of a breech is one of the nightmares of breech delivery.

> **If a grand multipara says that she wants to push, BELIEVE HER**, even if her cervix was only 3 cm dilated 5 minutes earlier. She will be fully dilated!

It is important to discuss future contraception *antenatally* as sterilization may be acceptable to her. However, the pressures of her large family waiting at home for her services will often lead her to decline the offer as she has not got the time to spare. The grand multipara, more than most patients, needs in-patient rest after delivery, family pressures permitting. Postpartum iron/folic acid therapy is also advisable.

Gross obesity

The grossly obese woman does not usually find that pregnancy is an enjoyable experience. Many minor ailments of pregnancy are increased.

General problems of obesity in pregnancy

- varicose veins
- haemorrhoids
- backache
- ankle oedema
- dyspnoea on effort
- intertrigo.

During pregnancy any positive weight-reducing plans should be abandoned temporarily. The expert help of a dietician is, however, invaluable.

Essential hypertension is far commoner in the obese woman. (A large cuff should always be used when taking the blood pressure, as a normal-sized cuff will give an inaccurately high reading.) If one can predict any one problem occuring during the pregnancy, it will be a need for admission because of super-imposed pregnancy-induced hypertension. There is also an association between hypertension and an increased risk of antepartum haemorrhage due to abruptio placentae.

Gross obesity is an indication to carry out a glucose tolerance test at 28 weeks in view of an increased tendency to develop gestational diabetes.

Antenatal problems assosciated with gross obesity

- all minor ailments increased
- essential hypertension
- pregnancy-induced hypertension
- gestational diabetes
- abruptio placentae.

The huge size of the maternal abdomen can make palpation a difficult exercise. Malpresentations may go unrecognized. The baby may be considerably larger than expected as its true size has been masked by the thickness of the surrounding maternal abdominal wall. Ultrasonography can be invaluable and should be readily available. Ultrasound estimations of fetal weight can be helpful and are likely to be more accurate than guesswork. When the baby is thought to be large, very careful pelvic assesment is necessary in the primigravida. Any incidental problem such as acute abdominal pain, which can be difficult enough to diagnose during pregnancy in the woman of normal weight, becomes a nightmare in the grossly obese.

Because of hypertensive complications, there is a greater need for labour to be induced. The sheer bulk of the patient can make access for pelvic examinations difficult. She will often find it difficult to become comfortable during labour.

Problems in labour associated with gross obesity

- difficulty in insertion of epidural block
- increased operative delivery
- postpartum haemorrhage.

Operative intervention, whether by forceps or Caesarean section, can be extremely difficult owing to problems of access.

When a postpartum haemorrhage occurs in the obese patient, it is definitely not the right time to try to find a vein for a drip! Have a drip up and running during labour.

Tissue healing is always a problem in the obese patient following surgery. Episiotomy and Caesarean scars can easily become infected and break down. Lying still in bed after delivery considerably increases the risk of thrombo-embolic disease.

Lactation is much more difficult to establish, with the result that attempts at breast-feeding are often abandoned.

The perinatal mortality rate among these women is significantly increased due to the higher incidence of hypertensive disorders and problems relating to labour.

The hugely obese woman in pregnancy is not a happy one. She needs considerable medical support. The time for tackling her weight problem is postpartum and her weight reduction must be closely supervised. Contraceptive advice is also essential so that she does at least have an opportunity to lose some of her bulk before returning to the antenatal clinic again.

Sterilization request

It is quite common for a woman to make a request for a sterilization at her first antenatal visit. There are obviously going to be a number of factors that will determine whether or not such a request is reasonable.

1. *The age of the patient and her partner*. Unless there are major medical reasons, it is generally unwise to agree to a sterilization being carried out on the very young woman. Bearing in mind that at least one in three marriages break down, it would be foolhardly to carry out such a final method of contraception when there are usually perfectly adequate alternatives.

2. *The number of children by her current partner*. If a woman has had children by a previous relationship, and this pregnancy is only going to be the first or second child by a new partner, it would be in her family's best interests to delay the sterilization until such a time as she is certain that her baby is thriving and less likely to succumb to Sudden Infant Death Syndrome ('cot death'). Even if this second child is to be delivered by an elective Caesarean section, the temptation to sterilize should be resisted. [Many patients are under the impression that they will not be allowed to have more than three Caesarean sections. The world record is 13!]

3. *Puerperal sterilization or interval sterilization?* Unless the family is large, and obviously complete, then it is reasonable to think in terms of puerperal sterilization (Table 2.2). Often the patient that the obstetrician is keenest to sterilize, such as the 'grand multip' with poor social circumstances, is the one who eventually will not be prepared to stay in hospital because of the demands made upon her by her large family.

Table 2.2 Advantages and disadvantages of puerperal versus interval sterilization

Puerperal	Interval
No opportunity to become pregnant after delivery	Will need adequate interim contraception
Mini-laparotomy and longer in-patient stay	Laparoscopy as a day case
Must run the gauntlet of 'cot death' risk	Will have passed risk of 'cot death'

It is essential to date and document all information that is given to a woman regarding sterilization. *The final decison should be made by a senior member of staff only.*

For example:

Date

(1) aware of finality of sterilization;

(2) appreciates the 1 in 600 failure rate of female sterilization;

(3) appreciates the higher success rate of vasectomy (only 1 in 5000 failure rate *after* two consecutive negative semen analyses have been obtained);

(4) aware of 1 in 500 'cot death' risk, chiefly in the first 6 months of life but up to 18 months.

DECISION:

signed

The worst time for a woman to come to a decision about sterilization is as she is being wheeled down the corridor for her emergency Caesarean section. Her overwhelming concern is for the welfare of her baby, and she is likely to agree to anything as long as her baby is safe. Even if it is her third Caesarean section, if she has not had a full opportunity to discuss and consider sterilization, *do not sterilize her*! A day-case laparoscopic sterilization can always be done at a later date.

Hasty decisions to sterilize are often regretted at leisure and may have medico-legal consequences.

Remember that a sterilization is quick and easy to do but may be difficult or impossible to reverse. If there is any doubt, keep her options open and defer the decision.

3   Antenatal problems

This section deals with the practical management of antenatal problems. For ease of reference, problems have been categorized into three sections:

(1) minor everyday complaints in pregnancy;
(2) antenatal complications;
(3) disorders and disease in pregnancy.

Minor everyday complaints in pregnancy

The majority of pregnant women will experience some minor 'nuisance' problems which can certainly reduce their sense of well-being. Many women will simply put up with these, being reluctant to appear to be making a fuss. An important role of every professional involved in antenatal care is to ensure that patients should never feel that they are wasting anybody's time by seeking reassurance, even if the problem proves to be only a trivial one. Sometimes it isn't. It is to be hoped the information given to them at the booking clinic, whether at the GP's surgery or the consultant unit, will encourage them always to seek medical advice.

Nausea and vomiting

While nausea and vomiting are very common symptoms of early pregnancy, their daily occurrence can turn the first trimester into an intensely miserable experience. Fortunately, these symptoms usually diminish considerably by the 16th week. Vomiting frequently occurs in the early morning but can occur at any time of the day. The majority of patients can achieve significant relief from these symptoms by dietary means. Small, frequent, non-fatty, dry, high-calorie meals, as opposed to the standard three main meals each day,is the simplest measure.

> **If vomiting is excessive in early pregnancy, the possibility of multiple pregnancy or hydatidiform mole must be kept in mind.**

There is an understandable reluctance by patients to take antiemetic drugs because of a fear of teratogenic effects. However, if symptoms do not settle with dietary adjustment, then medication *should* be given. The most commonly prescribed drugs that may be used with safety include:

- **promethazine** (Avomine, Phenergan) 25 mg tablet nocte and if required may be taken 8-hourly
- **prochlorperazine** (Stemetil) 5 mg tablet 8-hourly or as a suppository in the same dosage

It must be remembered that there are other causes of vomiting which may be unrelated to the pregnancy. These include gastroenteritis, appendicitis, acute pyelonephritis, and accidents to ovarian cysts and fibroids.

> **When marked vomiting occurs late in pregnancy, there is usually a significant pathological cause.**

It will occasionally happen that vomiting is so severe that even water cannot be retained and medications given as an out-patient appear to be useless. In that case, emergency admission is required (*see* hyperemesis gravidarum, p. 116).

> **The patient must be aware of the importance in seeking medical advice if vomiting becomes uncontrollable.**

Constipation

This common symptom in pregnancy is due to the muscle-relaxing effect of progesterone on the smooth muscle of the bowel. Dietary measures such as increasing the fibre content of meals, as well as the amount of fresh fruit, vegetables, and water, can be very effective.

When drugs are necessary it is preferable to use preparations that effectively add bulk to the stool and so increase peristalsis. Bulking agents are safe to use as they are not absorbed from the gastrointestinal tract:

- **lactulose solution BP** (Lactulose) 15 ml twice a day.
- **ispaghula husk** (Fybogel) 3.5 g sachet with water twice a day after meals.

Stool softeners can also be helpful:

- **Senna** (Senokot) 2 tablets or 5 ml granules or 10 ml syrup nocte.

Suppositories and enemas are rarely required except after surgery. Their action tends to be more vigorous than the above preparations. Very violent bowel movements can have an adverse effect on the neighbouring pregnant uterus.

> Enemas should never be used if a woman has threatened to miscarry or has a known placenta praevia.

Prophylactic iron preparations can exacerbate a woman's tendency to constipation. The form of iron may need to be changed or the amount taken reduced.

Heartburn

Heartburn of pregnancy is probably due to the smooth muscle-relaxing properties of progesterone upon the sphincters of the stomach. Reflux of acid gastric contents and bile irritates the lower oesophagus.

Simple measures such as small, frequent meals and sleeping in a more propped-up position can be helpful but are usually inadequate.

Antacid preparations or combination compounds also containing alginates can be very beneficial:

- **magnesium** and **aluminium hydroxides** (Maalox) 10 ml, 20 minutes after meals and nocte
- **sodium alginate** and **bicarbonate** with **calcium carbonate** (Gaviscon) 10 ml, 20 minutes after meals and nocte.

Varicose veins

Varicosities may either appear for the first time in pregnancy or, if pre-existing, may become worse. Increasing pelvic pressure from the growing uterus is the chief causative factor. Varicosities may appear in the legs, vulva, abdominal wall, and also as haemorrhoids.

Varicose veins in the legs are best controlled by means of support. If support tights or stockings are to be worn, these should be put on while the patient is still horizontal in bed and the veins are relatively collapsed. In hot weather such heavy support is uncomfortable to wear and keeping the legs elevated whenever possible is the only alternative solution.

Varicosities of the vulva can be very dramatic in appearance and alarm the patient. Apart from discomfort they do not cause a problem antenatally. Usually vulval varicosities only involve the labia but if they extend around to the introitus of the vagina or involve the perineum, problems could arise if an episiotomy is required at delivery. It is usually possible to direct the episiotomy away from the major varicosities. Vulval varicosities always slowly disappear after delivery.

Abdominal wall varicosities are unsightly but do not cause any problems. They disappear after delivery. Occasionally a patient will present with a large groin swelling in the third trimester caused by a varicocele of the round ligament of the uterus. This is invariably misdiagnosed as being an inguinal hernia, even though the presence of an enlarged uterus would make this a virtually impossible occurence. The patient can be reassured that it will disappear after delivery.

Haemorrhoids can become very troublesome and suppositories may be required to give symptomatic relief. It is important to avoid constipation. A thrombosed pile can be agonizingly painful. Local anaesthetic preparations are usually all that is required and it is rare that surgical intervention is necessary.

Backache

The commonest cause of back pain is the back itself. The centre of gravity in a non-pregnant woman will go through the knees, but the presence of a large anterior abdominal mass brings the centre of gravity forward, in front of the knees. To prevent herself from toppling forwards onto her face, every pregnant woman subconciously changes her posture by increasing lumbar lordosis. These changes, combined with relaxation of ligaments, lead to pressure on nerve roots and produce pain. If there has been a pre-existing back problem such as a disc prelapse, pregnancy can exacerbate the condition. Bed rest, increasing the firmness of the mattress with boards placed beneath it and, occasionally, a pregnancy supporting brace-girdle are the simplest remedies. Admission to hospital is rarely necessary.

Coccydynia should always thought of if a patient complains of severe 'tail-end' pain which may make normal sitting down an impossibility. If a rectal examination is performed with the patient in the left lateral position, the coccyx can be gently grasped between the examining finger and the external thumb. In coccydynia, the slightest movement of the coccyx on the sacro-coccygeal joint will cause exquisite pain. Analgesics are usually unhelpful. Many orthopaedic units run special coccydynia clinics. Intra-articular steroid/analgesic preparations can give profound relief.

Pelvic osteo-arthropathy

Under the influence of progesterone, the symphysis pubis will separate as pregnancy progresses. The resulting 'give' in the pelvis is desirable with regard to increasing the antero-posterior diameter available for the fetus to negotiate through. Occasionally the degree of pelvic 'opening' can be excessive, virtually amounting to a spontaneous symphysiotomy. Each half of the pelvis will move independently against the opposite half, producing severe pain over the symphysis and lower back. The gap in the symphysis will be pronounced and very tender to minimal pressure. The pain is exacerbated by asking the woman to stand on one leg, which causes the opposite side of the pelvis to drop. As a result, walking may be completely impossible. Bed rest in hospital may be necessary. Braced pelvic supports are available which can be very helpful. The condition slowly improves after delivery.

Carpal tunnel syndrome

Oedema beneath the flexor retinaculum of the wrist is a common occurrence, producing a tingling sensation in the fingers. When the oedema is severe enough to be able to compress the median nerve, the tingling increases to pain which can radiate up the forearm. The patient will often find that first thing in the morning she can hardly use her hand. The fingers feel stiff and useless and she will often drop things. If delivery is imminent, explanation and reassurance that the condition will be relieved almost immediately afterwards is usually sufficient. If delivery is still several weeks away, it is best to refer the to the woman to the surgical appliances department so that she can be fitted with 'night splints'. These dorsiflex the wrist and reduce the pressure on the median nerve. (It is worth while ordering two splints so that one can be washed while the other is being worn.)

Other common musculo-skeletal pains

Pain in one or both groin areas is commonly due to *stretching of the round ligaments* of the uterus as they pass to their labial insertion. The uterus itself is soft and not tender. Explanation of the probable cause of the pain is usually sufficient to relieve the understandable anxiety it can cause. Simple analgesics may be necessary.

Chest pain is always a worrying symptom to anyone experiencing it. Pleuritic-type pain may occur in late pregnancy in a patient who is otherwise well. It is usually due to the effect that the enlarging uterus has in elevating the diaphragm, and the subsequent alteration in the shape of the rib cage. Tenderness over the intercostal muscles at the site of the pain is common. Reassurance and simple analgesics are all that are required.

Vaginal discharge

The normal acidic environment of the vagina is very protective against ascending infection. This acidity is due to the action of Doderlein's bacilllus upon vaginal glycogen. Although in pregnancy there is an increase in the glycogen content of vaginal cells, the corresponding increase in vaginal acidity can be offset by a more profuse production of alkaline cervical mucus. As a result the woman may become aware of a clear/white vaginal discharge. If there is no offensive aroma, soreness, or pruritus vulvae, she may simply be reassured that her discharge is physiological and is of no significance.

However, the combination of a high glycogen content and warmth can be an ideal culture medium for certain pathogens in spite of the hostile acidity within the vagina.

Fungal infection with *Candida* species is very common in pregnancy. The discharge is generally thick and white and tends to adhere to the vaginal skin. There may or may not be associated pruritus vulvae. The diagnosis is confirmed either by taking a high vaginal swab for culture in the appropriate culture medium or by direct microscopy of the discharge.

The treatment of candida infections in pregnancy can be difficult, as clinical response tends to be slower and recurrences are commoner. It is, however, worth while to attempt to clear any candida infection even if repeated courses of treatment are required, both for the alleviation of symptoms and to prevent an oral candida infection in the baby. Systemic therapy is contraindicated in pregnancy and generally one of the topical imidazole preparations will be effective. The commonly used imidazoles include:

- **miconazole** (Gyno-Daktarin, Monistat)
- **clotrimazole** (Canesten)
- **econazole** (Gyno-Pevaryl, Ecostatin).

Depending upon the clinical situation and the preference of the clinician, these preparations may be given either as a vaginal pessary or in a cream form. Treatment may be prescribed as a single-dose pessary or as a 3–6 day course. When candida infections recur, it is important to give advice as to general hygiene and the abandoning of nylon gussetted tights and of poorly ventilated, tight-fitting clothing.

Infection with *Trichomonas vaginalis* produces intense pruritus vulvae and often a profuse green/yellow watery discharge. She may complain that intercourse is impossible. The diagnosis depends upon finding motile trichomonads within the discharge. A high vaginal swab should be taken for the laboratory. Treatment consists of prescribing metronidazole (Flagyl) 200 mg three times a day to *both* partners.

Gardnerella vaginalis infection produces a clear, offensive vaginal discharge, but only rarely is there a vulvitis (unlike candida and trichomonas infections). A high vaginal swab will easily pick up this infection. Treatment is the same as for trichomonas infection.

> It is tempting to guess at the cause of a vaginal discharge, and then be wrong. Send a high vaginal swab in culture medium to the laboratory.

Antenatal complications

Bleeding in early pregnancy

Bleeding, however slight, is always going to be a cause of anxiety to the pregnant woman. Most women know that such bleeding is abnormal and could indicate the beginning of a miscarriage process. All patients should be encouraged to report *any* vaginal bleeding immediately to their medical advisors.

> Even minimal bleeding is potentially serious and should be regarded as threatening the pregnancy and the well-being of the patient.

The woman will probably first contact her midwife or GP, although she may ring the hospital direct to seek advice and reassurance. If the bleeding has been minimal, is not continuing, and there is no associated pain, it is reasonable initially to simply advise complete bed rest at home until there has been no bleeding for 48 hours. Most GPs will have access to ultrasonography, which can be very reassuring to the patient. She can then gently mobilize herself. This is, of course, with the proviso that she seeks further immediate assistance if the bleeding should become heavier or any abdominal pain should occur. Sometimes the bleeding will be post-coital and a subsequent speculum examination may reveal a cervical polyp or cervical ectopy which bleeds on touch. She should be advised to abstain from intercourse or at least avoid deep penetration. In many cases of slight vaginal bleeding, no obvious cause is ever found and it does not recur.

If the bleeding is more than slight and especially if there is lower abdominal pain, then admission to hospital is advisable because of the risks associated with abortion. Very occasionally, the bleeding is so torrential that resuscitation in the patient's home is required before she is fit to be transferred into hospital. In such cases the obstetric 'flying squad' may need to be called out by the GP.

Abortion is defined as the termination of pregnancy before the 24th week and will occur in up to 25 per cent of all pregnancies. Classically, the patient will, after a variable period of amenorrhoea, present with vaginal bleeding. This may initially be slight, but with the development of uterine contractions, the blood loss increases, the cervix dilates and eventually the products of conception are completely or incompletely passed. The various types of spontaneous abortion simply reflect the stage reached in the abortion process.

When first admitted, the patient is usually distraught over the posibility that she may be about to lose her baby. It is very easy for the busy SHO having to admit several patients when 'on take', to rush through the business of clerking and examining the patient, tell her that she has lost the baby, get her to sign the consent form for an evacuation of her uterus, take some blood, and move on to the next patient. Clinically, all the medical moves will have been correct, except for the most important one, namely forgetting that an anguished woman has now been told that her pregnancy has ended. Just a few moments of time, caring, and sympathy can do much to prevent many months of anger directed at the medical profession for their inability to save her baby, long-term depression, bitterness, guilt, and even a sense of failure.

The initial diagnosis regarding the inevitability of an abortion will depend upon the clinical findings at pelvic examination. A speculum examination will allow inspection of the cervix. A bimanual examination of the uterus is of considerable value and *if carried out gently does not lead to abortion*. It is, however, wise to first inform the patient of this fact *before* a vaginal examination is performed. Otherwise, human nature being what it is, she will link the two events together. The aim of the bimanual examination is to assess the size of the uterus, its compatibility to her dates, and to exclude the presence of an adnexal swelling which may suggest the diagnosis of an ectopic pregnancy.

Threatened abortion

A closed cervix does not necessarily mean that all is well, but at least implies that the abortion process may not yet be inevitable. A diagnosis of threatened abortion is made. The treatment is bed rest until there has been no vaginal loss for 48 hours. Each morning on getting up for toilet purposes, the patient may be disconcerted to notice an apparent increase in dark brown blood-stained discharge, but this may simply be due to the drainage of old blood into the upper vagina which only becomes apparent when she is vertical and the loss can drain more easily. During this resting stage a daily ward pregnancy test should be performed and ultrasonography arranged. If she is only 6–7 weeks pregnant by dates (especially after adjusting for an irregular cycle), it would not be expected to see fetal heart movements, except by vaginal ultrasound.

> Beware the diagnosis of 'probable incomplete abortion' made at ultrasonography in very early pregnancy. Frequently, a repeat scan a week or two later will reveal fetal heart movements.

The serial quantitative measurements of hCG can be helpful in the management of early threatened abortions, as during the first 6 weeks of pregnancy the β-hCG level doubles every 48 hours. Thereafter, there is a slower steady increase, reaching a peak which can be as high as 300 000 IU/l by 13 weeks. This then falls by mid-pregnancy to settle around 50 000 IU/l. Once the β-hCG level reaches 6000 IU/l there should be ultrasound evidence of a pregnancy. If not, laparoscopy is indicated to exclude an ectopic pregnancy. A rapidly falling β-hCG below 6000 IU/l probably indicates that the pregnancy will fail. If the β-hCG is less than 5 IU/l an ongoing pregnancy is excluded but does not rule out the possibility of a recent intrauterine pregnancy or an ectopic that has aborted.

Once fetal heart movements are seen and all bleeding and pain have ceased for 48 hours, the woman can be mobilized and if still asymptomatic may be discharged home to rest. She should be advised to abstain from intercourse. Follow-up in the antenatal clinic is arranged.

As a general rule, the heavier the bleeding, the greater the likelihood of an inevitable abortion.

Inevitable abortion

If, on admission with bleeding and painful contractions, the cervix is found to be dilating, a diagnosis of inevitable abortion is made. The pregnancy cannot be salvaged by any form of treatment. On bimanual examination, it is not always possible to diagnose whether or not the abortion process is **complete** with all products of conception having been passed, or **incomplete**, with some products of conception being retained within the uterus. If bleeding is minimal and the cervix is dilated, it is reasonable to await the results of ultrasound scanning which will show if there are retained products within the uterine cavity.

Frequently, clot and products of conception may be seen distending the cervical canal. It is worth while gently removing products from the cervical canal with sponge holders, as this simple manoeuvre can considerably reduce the amount of pain, bleeding, and shock experienced by the patient.

If the cervix is dilated and the bleeding is heavy, there is little point in waiting for ultrasound confirmation of the diagnosis. There will be retained products or at least a considerable amount of retained clot, which to all intents and purposes is the same thing. An intravenous infusion needs to be set up, blood taken for grouping and save-serum or cross-matching, and intravenous ergometrine 0.25–0.5 mg administered. An evacuation of retained products of conception is arranged. Torrentially heavy vaginal bleeding in the aborting patient is an emergency and evacuation of the uterus is a matter of urgency, regardless of the time of day or night, the anaesthetist's worry about the patient's recent meal, or even the prior claims of general surgeons with a ?appendicitis patient. If diplomacy is unsuccessful in obtaining prompt theatre space, the additional clout of a senior member of the team will be required! If bleeding is minimal, it is reasonable to carry out the evacuation on the next emergency operating list, e.g. the next morning if the patient has been admitted after midnight.

It should be remembered that until relatively recently, abortion was the major cause of maternal death, due to haemorrhage, infection, and shock.

In the Report on Confidential Enquiries into Maternal Deaths in the UK (1988–90), 6.2 per cent (nine cases) of all direct deaths were due to abortion.

Septic abortion

On admission, some aborting patients are found to be febrile, with a tender uterus and an offensive vaginal loss. The abortion process has, therefore, become septic. Swabs should be taken for culture. If the temperature is high, blood cultures are also advisable. Antibiotic therapy in high dosage is essential. Combinations of intravenous antibiotics are usual:

- **ampicillin** 1 g initially IV and then 500 mg four times a day *or*
- **cefuroxime** 1.5 g initially IV and then 0.75 g three times a day *and*
- **metronidazole** 500 mg IV three times a day.

If bleeding is not heavy, it is reasonable to delay the evacuation of the uterus for 24 hours to allow the operation to be performed under the 'antibiotic umbrella'.

> Heavy vaginal bleeding must be stopped even in the presence of major infection. The uterine evacuation is carried out as a matter of urgency.

Evacuation of retained products can be difficult even for the experienced operator. The pregnant uterus is much softer than in the non-pregnant state and perforation is relatively easy. Sometimes the retrieval of products seems to be endless. Rather than to persist with the operation and perforate the uterus, it is better to stop and return the patient to the ward, and possibly have to repeat the curettage a day or two later.

The Confidential Enquiries into Maternal Deaths reported that 6 of the 9 women mentioned above died as a result of sepsis. The Report highlighted substandard care due largely to the absence of consultation between junior and senior medical staff and the failure to refer serious problems early enough to ITU. Even in critical situations junior staff were failing to seek help or advice.

> NEVER hesitate in seeking help from senior staff.

A patient who miscarries will often be admitted, have her evacuation of retained products, and be discharged within 24 hours. One moment she is happily looking forward to the outcome of her pregnancy, and the next moment there is nothing. Do not underestimate the profound emotional stress that this can cause both partners. Trite comments such as 'Nature know, best' and 'Better luck next time' are not helpful. She must be given the opportunity to ask questions and receive answers. If she has had recurrent abortions (**habitual abortion**) she should be followed up in the gynaecological out-patient or infertility clinic. It is also very helpful to many couples to be given the address of the Miscarriage Association which can be immensely supportive and informative.

Missed abortion

A missed abortion does not cause bleeding in early pregnancy until it is eventually expelled by the uterus. It is, however, included in this section for completeness. It is generally first suspected in the antenatal clinic because the uterus is considerably smaller than expected dates. Subsequent ultrasonography shows either an empty gestation sac ('blighted ovum') or a fetus without any visible heart movements. If there is no bleeding, many patients will prefer to wait and have the scan repeated before finally agreeing to have the uterus emptied. If bleeding should occur during this 'waiting interval', she must be advised to be immediately admitted to hospital. There is the risk of clotting disorders in the patient if the evacuation is delayed for several weeks. Fortunately, this complication is rarely seen. If the uterus is smaller than 12–14 weeks in size it can be safely evacuated using suction curettage. The larger uterus will require an 'induction of labour' with prostaglandins initially and possibly oxytocin later. Once the pregnancy has been aborted, an evacuation of retained products is usually necessary.

> In the rhesus-negative patient, it is essential that anti-D immunoglobulin is administered to prevent rhesus iso-immunization.

Hydatidiform mole

Bleeding in early pregnancy, associated with hyperemesis, a uterus large for dates (although not necessarily so) and, especially, early signs of fulminating pre-eclampsia, must suggest the diagnosis of a hydatidiform mole. On examination, no fetal heart can be heard using an ultrasound fetal heart detector. Ultrasonography shows a characteristic 'snowstorm' appearance which fills the uterus with echoes. Urinary pregnancy tests will be positive in dilutions of more than 1 in 200 owing to the very high levels of hCG. The passage of grape-like vesicles is absolutely diagnostic.

Once the diagnosis has been reached, the uterus must be evacuated. This can be a haemorrhagic procedure and at least 2 units of blood should be cross-matched and available in the theatre.

> These patients can bleed ferociously. The evacuation should always be by means of suction curettage and only be carried out by an experienced operator.

If there is any doubt over the completeness of the evacuation, a curettage 2 weeks later is strongly recommended. This relatively rare condition will affect 1 in 2000 pregnancies in western countries, but is three times commoner in the Far East.

Once the histology is obtained, the patient must be referred to the supra-regional endocrine assay department for monitoring for up to 2 years, as there is the possibility of subsequent malignant trophoblastic disease in the form of a **choriocarcinoma** in 2–3 per cent of cases. During the monitoring period, contraception should continue. A rise in hCG levels could be the first sign of a choriocarcinoma but could also simply be due to a normal pregnancy.

Ectopic pregnancy

An extrauterine pregnancy is a relatively common cause of pain and bleeding in early pregnancy.

Ectopic pregnancy is a potentially fatal condition, so early diagnosis is of the utmost importance.

In the Report on Confidential Enquiries into Maternal Deaths in the UK (1988–90), ectopic pregnancy is the fourth major cause (10.3 per cent) of all direct deaths after hypertension, pulmonary embolism, and haemorrhage from other causes. In the report there were 19 ectopic deaths, 15 (79 per cent) occuring as a direct result of rupturing of the ectopic pregnancy. Seven of the 15 deaths were considered to involve substandard care.

There is no difficulty in diagnosing the classic textbook case. The patient presents with a history of amenorrhoea of more than 4 weeks duration (thereby raising the possibility of a pregnancy), lower abdominal pain, and a dark brown, blood-stained vaginal discharge or moderate bleeding. On direct questioning she may admit to having felt faint or dizzy on standing or an sitting up from a lying-down position, and to have experienced shoulder-tip pain. On examination, there may be tenderness in the lower abdomen. On gentle bimanual, vaginal exami-nation, the cervix may be soft and a tender pulsatile mass may be felt through one of the lateral fornices of the vagina.

A ruptured ectopic pregnancy presents with no diagnostic problems. The patient will be collapsed with a rapid pulse, a low and possibly unmeasure-able blood pressure and a distended abdomen full of blood (*see* Antenatal emergencies).

The problem with ectopic pregnancy is that it does not always oblige by presenting in the classical manner. The most common misdiagnosis is of a threatened abortion. The patient may have a history of amenorrhoea and a positive pregnancy test, with recent vaginal bleeding and pain and no other symptoms of note. A speculum examination is not particularly helpful in establishing the diagnosis, as an adnexal swelling will be missed. It is for this reason that a gentle bimanual examination (once the patient is in the safe environment of a hospital) is important when a patient presents as a threatened abortion.

> Ectopic pregnancies tend to present with '*p*' *p*ain before bleeding whereas abortion will present with '*b*' *b*leeding before pain.

The patient may have irregular periods and not present with any amenorrhoea of note. She may only be complaining of slight vaginal bleeding and pain. In spite of being afebrile, chronic pelvic inflammatory disease is frequently diagnosed, especially if there is a recent history of having had an IUCD (intrauterine contraceptive device) inserted or removed. Pelvic tenderness may be vague and no adnexal mass may be felt.

> Unilateral pelvic tenderness does not occur in acute pelvic inflammatory disease. An ectopic pregnancy must be excluded.

Even an experienced gynaecologist will occasionally miss an ectopic pregnancy. A diagnosis of incomplete abortion may be made and an evacuation of retained products of conception carried out. The clue to the true diagnosis becomes apparent from the histology report of the so-called 'products of conception'. There will be no chorionic villi present but only a marked decidual reaction. Unless there is a history of a fetus having been passed, such a report would be an indication to recall the patient urgently.

> ALWAYS send retained products of conception for histology. Even obvious placental remnants may turn out to be decidua only.

Awareness of the possibility of an ectopic pregnancy must always be in the forefront of the admitting doctor's conciousness. Experience dictates that it is sensible to regard every emergency admission of a woman of reproductive age as pregnant until proven otherwise. When there are symptoms of bleeding or pain, the site of that pregnancy must also be suspect until proven to be intra-uterine. THINK ECTOPIC!

> The early diagnosis of ectopic pregnancy is essential and can be lifesaving. When there is difficulty in making the diagnosis, ALWAYS seek senior medical help and advice.

Certain patient groups in particular should alert the clinician as to the true diagnosis when they present with an atypical history:

(1) a previous ectopic pregnancy;

(2) a recent history of an IUCD insertion or removal;

(3) a past history of pelvic inflammatory disease;

(4) tubal surgery for infertility;

(5) the sterilized patient.

> If an ectopic pregnancy is suspected, it must be excluded *before* discharging the patient home.

A positive pregnancy test, adnexal pain, and a palpable adnexal mass, indicates the need for an urgent laparoscopy to establish the diagnosis.

> A negative pregnancy test does not rule out the possibility of an ectopic pregnancy.

Apart from laparoscopy, the two most important investigations are the beta-hCG estimation and ultrasonography.

A raised beta-hCG indicates the presence of a pregnancy somewhere, but in itself can give no suggestion as to the site of that pregnancy. Once the beta-hCG reaches 6000 IU/l, a gestation sac should be visible within the uterus on ultrasonography and, if not seen, indicates the need for laparoscopy. At lower levels of beta-hCG, ultrasound may reveal the presence of an adnexal swelling, again indicating the need for laparoscopy. The absence of an adnexal mass at ultrasound does not rule out a diagnosis of ectopic pregnancy. Similarly, a normal (non-pregnant) level of beta-hCG may be associated with a tubal abortion.

A raised beta-hCG and unilateral adnexal tenderness in a patient complaining of pain and/or vaginal bleeding MUST be regarded as indicating an ectopic pregnancy until proven otherwise.

Once the diagnosis of a probable ectopic pregnancy has been made, it is important that the diagnosis is confirmed by laparoscopy as a matter of urgency. An intravenous infusion should be set up and blood sent for cross-matching. The patient must understand the nature of her possible condition and the need for laparotomy and possible removal of the Fallopian tube if the diagnosis is confirmed. It is not wise to delay these cases to the next morning's operating list. Such lists have the habit of developing their own problems, necessitating the further delay of the laparoscopy. Operating at night when there are no pressures from other list cases is preferable to waiting and risking the rupture of an ectopic. When an ectopic pregnancy ruptures, the change in the patient's well-being is dramatic.

The collapsed patient from a ruptured ectopic must be resuscitated and taken directly to theatre. The involment of medical expertise cannot be over-stressed. The combination of a senior anaesthetist, gynaecologist, and haematologist is essential to prevent disaster. *Early* adequate blood transfusion is imperative as well as central venous pressure (CVP) monitoring to prevent over-transfusion and pulmonary oedema.

Unless vaginal bleeding is heavy, there is no need to carry out a curettage at the time of laparoscopy, as occasionally there can be an ongoing intrauterine pregnancy in association with the ectopic. For this reason it is also best initially not to cannulate the uterus. If there is a large amount of clot present in the pelvis at laparoscopy, the diagnosis is virtually certain and an immediate laparotomy is performed. It is far safer to remove the severely ruptured tube *even if it is the only tube she has left*. There may always be the possible option of a future attempt at *in vitro* fertilization.

If the tube has not ruptured, *and depending on the health of the contralateral tube*, salpingotomy and simply leaving the tube open after removing the ectopic, is preferable to salpingectomy, as even the tube which has had one ectopic pregnancy within it in the past, does have the potential of permitting an intra-uterine pregnancy to occur on a subsequent occasion. (Many gynaecologists will feel that if the tube is conserved one is simply begging for another ectopic. However, there is a 10 per cent chance of another ectopic occuring in the remaining tube, so the risk is still present.) 'Milking' an ectopic from the ampulla of the tube tends to cause bleeding and requires haemostatic manoeuvres which can result in the loss of the tube.

Remember always to check the opposite tube. One in 650 ectopics is bilateral!

Minimally invasive surgery is playing an increasingly large part in the management of ectopic pregnancy. This requires the proper training of both the medical and theatre nursing staff. At laparoscopy it is possible to remove even litres of clot, open the tube, remove the ectopic, and diathermy the base of the tube or any bleeding points. If it should prove to be necessary to remove the tube itself, this does not present major problems to the endoscopist.

Incidental bleeding

It is quite common to find some degree of **cervical ectopy** ('erosion'), or a **cervical polyp** on routine speculum examination at the antenatal booking clinic. If detected, it is best to simply advise the woman of the existence of the condition and that intercourse with deep penetration should be avoided. An episode of post-coital bleeding can cause considerable alarm to the couple unless they are warned from the outset that this can occur. There is rarely any need to treat either of these conditions before delivery.

Frank **cervical carcinoma** is a rare complication in pregnancy, affecting 1 in 3000 pregnancies. Unless a speculum and/or a bimanual examination are carried out at the booking assessment it may be missed. The treatment of this condition is no different from that in the non-pregnant state. If an invasive carcinoma is found before the 28th week, the pregnancy is sacrificed and surgery/radiotherapy is carried out. If the pregnancy has reached 28 weeks, it would not be unreasonable to allow a few weeks' grace to give the baby additional maturity and deliver by Caesarean section at 34 weeks. A subsequent Wertheim's hysterectomy could be carried out with or without radiotherapy.

For a summary of the causes any bleeding in early pregnancy, refer to Table 3.1.

Cervical incompetence

When an antenatal patient presents with a past history of a second trimester abortion, it is important to obtain as much information as possible about the incident, as this complication can recur. Once fetal abnormality, intrauterine death, infection, and multiple pregnancy have been excluded as predisposing causes, cervical incompetence and uterine anomalies such as a bicornuate uterus must be considered.

Table 3.1 Summary of causes of bleeding in early pregnancy

Abortion	
Spontaneous:	• threatened
	• inevitable
	• incomplete
	• complete
	• septic
	• missed
	• hydatidiform mole
Induced:	• therapeutic
	• criminal
Ectopic pregnancy	
Cervical pathology:	• cervical ectopy
	• cervical polypii
	• cervical carcinoma

> The cervix only begins to bear the weight of a pregnancy after the 15th week. Spontaneous abortions which occur before this gestation are unlikely to be due to an incompetent cervix.

A typical history of cervical incompetence will be of a patient more than 15 weeks pregnant, who experiences a sensation of fullness in the pelvis, followed by spontaneous rupture of the membranes and a short and relatively painless labour. If the actual abortion process has been preceded by several weeks of intermittent pain and bleeding, or if the abortion process itself is drawn-out and painful, then cervical incompetence is unlikely to be the cause.

Clinical examination may, or may not, be helpful. A short, patulous cervix that admits a finger confirms the diagnosis of cervical incompetence, but the converse is not true.

> The finding of a long, closed cervix does not exclude the possibility of cervical incompetence. If the history of the previous mid-trimester abortion is classical, *believe it*.

Where there is doubt, a weekly ultrasound scan after the 15th week can measure the length and degree of dilatation of the cervical canal. If, however, the history is clear-cut, the insertion of a cervical suture is indicated.

The insertion of a cervical 'circumsuture' can be extraordinarily difficult, especially if the cervix is very short. It may be performed either under general anaesthesia or a regional block such as an epidural anaesthetic. It is always helpful if, after the 3 mm mersilene tape suture has been tied, for a loop of the tape to be left tied onto the knot, so that there is something to grasp when the time comes for the eventual removal of the tape. (As the person who will one day need to remove the suture may not be the operator who inserted it, it is important that a clear description/diagram is put into the notes.)

Postoperatively, it is best to keep the patient on complete bed rest and mild sedation for 48 hours to reduce to a minimum the chances of abortion. Beta-sympathomimetic drugs such as ritodrine and salbutamol may also be indicated.

The woman must fully understand the need for immediate admission if she has any contractions or other signs of labour commencing while the suture is still in position.

> For medico-legal reasons, all cautionary information given to the patient must be entered into the notes, dated, and signed.

If she does not go into spontaneous labour, it is usual to remove the suture at 37 weeks, which will reduce the chances of the suture tearing through the cervix. Usually no anaesthetic is required. It is a simple matter to gently examine the patient vaginally, grasp the loop of mersilene tape with sponge-holding forceps, and cut the tape above the knot. Occasionally the cervix will immediately dilate.

> In true cervical incompetence, labour can be extraordinarily fast and precipitate.

If the cervix does not dilate, the woman should be returned to the ward, and be normally mobile until the next day, when she should be re-examined. If the cervix has still failed to dilate, she can be allowed to go home. She must, however, be told to return promptly at the first sign of labour commencing.

When a woman presents in the antenatal clinic with a history of recurrent abortions which are not typical of cervical incompetence, there is no point in inserting a suture. Close antenatal supervision is essential, with serial ultrasonography to monitor the pregnancy. There is a very real place for antenatal admission, especially to cover the weeks when she had previously aborted. Should she be unfortunate enough to abort again, she must be strongly advised not to get pregnant again until she has been fully assessed and investigated. These investigations will include hormonal assessment (does she have polycystic ovarian disease with high levels of luteinizing hormone?), glucose tolerance test, karyotyping of both partners, hysterosalpingography, hysteroscopy, and laparoscopy.

Anaemia in pregnancy

Iron-deficiency anaemia

During pregnancy, the circulating plasma volume increases by some 30 per cent, whereas the red cell mass only increases by 25 per cent. The resulting physiological anaemia is not harmful. However, it is generally recognized that the iron demands in pregnancy are greater than the iron saved by the absence of 9 months of menstruation. An iron-deficiency anaemia (haemoglobin less than 10 g/dl) commonly results. The arguments for and against prophylactic iron therapy have been discussed on p. 21. There are a number of proprietary brands of ferrous iron combined with folic acid that are taken on a once-a-day basis.

Severe iron-deficiency anaemia (haemoglobin less than 9 g/dl) must be adequately treated before delivery. If left untreated, the risk to both mother and baby is increased. The woman is unable to withstand blood loss in labour and perinatal mortality rate is doubled.

A falling haemoglobin level, in spite of oral iron therapy, *must* be investigated.

Investigations include:

- full blood count and film
- serum iron
- iron-binding capacity   } or serum ferritin
- serum B$_{12}$ and folate
- electrophoresis.

The haematological features of an iron-deficiency anaemia

haemoglobin ↓
mean corpuscular volume (MCV) ↓
mean corpuscular haemoglobin concentration (MCHC) ↓
serum iron ↓
iron-binding capacity ↑
serum ferritin ↓

There is no evidence that giving 'double iron' will speed up haemoglobin production. If there is an iron absorption problem, double oral iron will not help. (In the presence of a haemoglobinopathy, such as thalassaemia, excess iron administration may lead to haemosiderosis.)

Do not forget other sources of iron loss such as bleeding haemorrhoids, peptic ulcers, and bowel parasites. Iron deficiency is also associated with chronic urinary tract infection.

If the haemoglobin level fails to rise in spite of adequate oral iron therapy, parenteral therapy is indicated, as there is likely to be a problem with iron absorption from the bowel. The commonest form of parenteral iron therapy is an iron–sorbitol–citric acid complex (Jectofer) given by deep intramuscular injections into the buttock. A test dose must first be given. A course of 10 injections of 2 ml given on alternate days is adequate in the majority of cases. These injections are painful and will stain the skin unless administered by a Z-technique. (The skin of the buttock at the injection site is put 'on the stretch' as the injection is given. After injecting the Jectofer, the buttock skin is released so that the needle pathway on withdrawal is tortuous and so avoids tattooing the skin at the puncture site.) Iron is no longer administered intravenously as a total-dose infusion, owing to the considerable risk of fatal anaphylactic reactions.

If very severe anaemia only becomes apparent close to term, there will be insufficient time for any route of iron therapy to take effect before delivery. In such cases, blood transfusion will be the only way of ensuring a safe level of haemoglobin prior to the onset of labour. Every unit of packed cells will increase the haemoglobin by 1 g/dl.

[When anaemia is associated with poor diet and low socio-economic groups, it is advisable to recommend long-term oral iron therapy after delivery.]

Folate-deficiency anaemia

Folate-deficiency anaemia is not very common and rare amongst women who are taking a prophylactic iron/folic acid preparation. In pregnancy folate requirements are increased for DNA synthesis and the woman's normal diet may be deficient. Folate demands in a multiple pregnancy are obviously greater than for the singleton.

The haematological features of a folate-deficiency anaemia will include:

- haemoglobin ↓
- mean corpuscular volume (MCV) ↑
- mean corpuscular haemoglobin concentration (MCHC) ↓
- serum iron ↑↓
- serum folate ↓

The blood film should show macrocytic red cells and hypersegmented white cells. If there is any doubt about the diagnosis, the haematologist may recommend a bone marrow examination.

The treatment of folate deficiency is oral folic acid tablets 5–10 mg daily. While an iron-deficiency anaemia can coexist with a folate deficiency, the serum iron is usually high and no iron therapy is required.

Vitamin B_{12} deficiencies causing macrocytic anaemia are rarely seen in antenatal clinics as this condition tends to arise in an older age group.

Haemoglobinopathies

All patients of Mediterranean origin or from the Asian subcontinent should have an electrophoresis at booking to exclude beta-thalassaemia trait. All Afro-Caribbean women require sickle-cell screening to be performed. If a haemoglobinopathy is found, the partner's blood should also be checked. If the partner is also a carrier of the same condition, then antenatal diagnosis of the haematological status of the fetus is indicated. Chorionic villus sampling will provide tissue for DNA analysis. Cordocentesis later in pregnancy will provide an adequate fetal blood sample for diagnosis.

Heterozygous beta-thalassaemia (beta-thalassaemia trait) causes a mild chronic anaemia. Iron should be witheld unless there is evidence of a definite iron deficiency. Homozygous beta-thalassaemia causes such severe anaemia in childhood that death usually results and survival to adult life and pregnancy does not arise. However, there are many forms of beta-thalassaemia and some of these can be extremely mild.

Homozygous alpha-thalassaemia usually results in a hydropic fetus and stillbirth. These pregnancies are also complicated by pregnancy-induced hypertension and a considerable risk of postpartum haemorrhage due to massive placental hypertrophy.

Heterozygous sickle-cell disease (sickle-cell trait) does not cause serious problems to the pregnant woman. It is important that an anaesthetist is aware of the diagnosis as low oxygen tension can trigger off the sickling process.

Homozygous sickle-cell disease in pregnancy is associated with high maternal mortality and considerably increased perinatal mortality. Sickle-cell crisis results in severe bone pain, due to infarcts in bone, and an increased risk of thrombosis. Treatment consists of high dosages of folic acid, exchange transfusion of packed cells if there is a dramatic fall in haemoglobin, and heparin which reduces both the bone pain and the risk of thrombosis and embolism.

Among the Asian and Oriental community there is also a possibility of finding haemoglobin E thalassaemia, which results from a combination of haemoglobin E from one parent and beta-thalassaemia from another. There may be further complex problems, such as when one parent has sickle-cell trait and the other has beta-thalassaemia trait and the baby is at risk of having sickle-cell thalassaemia.

When these potential complex problems are found as a result of screening both parents, there must be close communication between obstetrician and haematologist. It is essential that expert genetic counselling is sought.

Disorders and disease in pregnancy

Urinary tract infections

In pregnancy, the tendency to develop urinary stasis increases the incidence of urinary tract infection (UTI). Six per cent of women have **asymptomatic bacteriuria**, where there are more than 100 000 bacteria per ml of urine in a mid-stream urine sample. The only way to detect this condition is to routinely carry out a urine culture at the booking appointment of every new antenatal patient.

The chief problems associated with asymptomatic bacteriuria

- acute pyelonephritis
- premature labour
- anaemia (due to reduced erythropoetin production).

Treatment is important, as 30 per cent of patients with asymptomatic bacteriuria will subsequently develop acute pyelonephritis. Fifty per cent of the patients who develop acute pyelonephritis will have had asymptomatic bacteriuria.

An appropriate course of an antibiotic is given. The choice of antibiotics is usually from ampicillin or amoxycillin, a cephalosporin, nitrofurantoin, and trimethoprin. Two weeks after treatment, a repeat urine sample is cultured, as the condition can recur in 35 per cent of cases. Should this occur, a course of different suitable antibiotic is given.

> Recurrent episodes of asymptomatic bacteriuria suggests a chronic renal condition such as chronic pyelonephritis, staghorn calculus, or anomalies of the bladder or ureters.

Patients who have recurrent infection must have a full investigation of the renal tract 3 months after delivery, by means of intravenous urography (IVU), by which time the ureteric dilatation caused by progesterone will have disappeared.

When an acute infection is confined to the bladder, the classic symptoms are of frequency, urgency, and dysuria. If infection involves the kidneys and ureters, pyrexia, rigors, vomiting, and loin pain are the presenting features.

All UTIs must be treated vigorously so as to reduce the risk of permanent renal damage. Ampicillin is effective in the majority of cases, and should be commenced without waiting for the antibiotic sensitivities. If necessary, the antibiotic can be changed once the sensitivities are available. A high fluid intake is important.

In acute pyelonephritis, the high temperature that commonly occurs must rapidly be brought under control as this is poorly tolerated by the baby and can even cause intrauterine death. Repeated tepid sponging will achieve this until antibiotic therapy becomes effective. Intravenous fluids are usually required to maintain intake owing to vomiting.

Repeated urine cultures should be carried out for the duration of the pregnancy, as the recurrence rate is high. Several courses of antibiotics may be required.

Hypertensive disorders in pregnancy

> At least 10 per cent of all pregnancies in the UK are complicated by hypertension.

Hypertension may either preceed pregnancy (essential hypertension) or arise as a result of the pregnancy itself (pregnancy-induced hypertension or pre-eclampsia). If the woman is known to have been hypertensive before pregnancy or is found to have a persistently raised blood pressure greater than 140/90 before the 20th week of pregnancy, it is reasonable to make a diagnosis of essential hypertension. If she has been normotensive during the first 20 weeks and only subsequently develops hypertension, then a diagnosis of pregnancy-induced hypertension is made. However, the label given to the type of hypertension may not always be as clear-cut as this.

Essential hypertension

Ten per cent of all pregnant hypertensive patients will be diagnosed as having essential hypertension.

The condition is commoner in the older woman (over 30) and there is usually a significant family history of hypertension.

When a persistently raised blood pressure is found *before 20 weeks in the younger woman*, other causes of hypertension must be excluded:

- chronic renal disease
- renal artery stenosis
- coarctation of the aorta
- phaeochromocytoma.

From the onset of pregnancy the effect of essential hypertension will be to reduce placental bed perfusion. The hypertension may worsen during the pregnancy, especially during the third trimester. Intrauterine growth retardation will therefore be the likely consequence.

Management
Once a diagnosis of essential hypertension has been made, the bulk of the antenatal care, especially after the 24th week, should be carried out by the consultant unit.

If her diastolic blood pressure remains below 100 mm Hg, the woman may be monitored as an out-patient. Some hospitals are fortunate in having an antenatal assessment area where accurate blood pressure monitoring and cardiotocography can be carried out on a regular basis. General advice should be given on diet, and the importance of adequate rest.

The basis of management of essential hypertension

(1) serial ultrasound scans
   biparietal diameter
   abdominal circumference
   fetal weight
   liquor volume;

(2) serial urate measurements at each antenatal visit;

(3) look out for proteinuria.

(4) antenatal cardiotocography;

(3) kick chart.

In cases of mild essential hypertension, the aim will be to deliver between 38 weeks and term.

When the diastolic blood pressure is 100 mmHg or above, admission is indicated in order to assess the need for hypotensive therapy. DO NOT COMMENCE HYPOTENSIVE THERAPY AS AN OUT-PATIENT.

When the patient has been admitted to the ward, the following are required:

- bed rest
- 4-hourly blood pressure recording
- daily cardiotocography
- and as above for mild essential hypertension.

> If the diastolic blood pressure does not settle below 100 mmHg, hypotensive therapy is conmenced. The aim of treatment is to keep the diastolic blood pressure at 90 mmHg or below.

Methyl dopa 250 mg three times a day increasing to a maximum of 750 mg four times a day. (This is the commonest hypotensive agent used by obstetricians.) Methyl dopa takes 2–3 days to become effective. Patients may complain of some sedative effect.

Labetalol 100 mg twice a day to 200 mg four times a day. There is evidence that this combined alpha and beta blocker is a better placental perfusor than beta blockers alone (such as atenolol and propranolol), and as such will increase placental bed blood flow and lead to an increase in fetal growth.

Hydralazine 10–20 mg intravenously is reserved for severe hypertensive states when the diastolic blood pressure is above 110 mmHg.

> Diuretics are contraindicated as they will only reduce the circulating blood volume and so reduce placental bed perfusion even further.

As long as the blood pressure is controlled, delivery should be planned for 38 weeks. A vaginal delivery can be carried out *as long as there are no additional complicating factors*, e.g. elderly primigravida, breech presentation. An epidural block is indicated for blood pressure control and analgesia.

When there is evidence of severe intrauterine growth retardation (especially if there are the added complications of impaired renal function and/or superimposed pregnancy-induced hypertension), it is generally safer to deliver the baby, *regardless of the gestational age*. Delivery of a small growth-retarded baby by elective Caesarean section means that the baby will be spared from having to face the stresses of labour as well as the problems of its prematurity. The safest policy must be to hand the baby over to the paediatricians in the best possible condition.

It is important to involve the woman and her partner in the discussion of the balance of risks. The problem of trying to buy time is to risk an intrauterine death. The problem of an early delivery is prematurity.

> REMEMBER that a paediatrician can usually do something to help a live baby. Nothing can be done to help a dead one!

Postnatally, every woman with essential hypertension must have medical follow-up to ensure that there is adequate supervision and control of her condition. If there has been no impairment of renal function, and her diastolic blood pressure remains below 100 mmHg, there is every prospect that a future pregnancy will be successful. Renal damage and a non-pregnancy diastolic blood pressure over 100 mmHg implies a poor outlook for any further pregnancy.

Pregnancy-induced hypertension (pre-eclampsia)

In the Report on Confidential Enquiries into Maternal Deaths in the UK (1988–90), hypertensive deaths are the major cause of maternal mortality. Pregnancy-induced hypertension (pre-eclampsia) and eclampsia were the sole cause of death in all 27 cases. Substandard care was significant in 88 per cent of cases. This was due to a combination of delayed medical intervention, poor control of the hypertension, and inappropriate responsibility given to junior medical staff.

Ninety per cent of all cases of hypertension in pregnancy will have pregnancy-induced hypertension (PIH).

The causes of PIH have only recently begun to be understood. Essentially, there is a failure of the trophoblast to completely invade and thereby destroy the muscle of the spiral arteries by the 22nd week. Therefore, the normal physiological dilatation of the spiral arteries, and the resulting falls in both the peripheral resistance and blood pressure, do not occur. The incompletely destroyed muscle coats of the spiral arteries retain their sensitivity to angiotensin II and undergo vasospasm. The further developments of atherosis, platelet aggregation, and eventual occlusion of the spiral arteries lead to an increase in peripheral resistance. The combinaton of the increased peripheral resistance and the expansion of the circulating blood volume in pregnancy produces a rise in blood pressure. The reduction in platelet bed perfusion and often gross placental infarction, causes intrauterine growth retardation and even intrauterine fetal death. The **platelet aggregation** and **disseminated intravascular coagulation (DIC)** can result in a coagulopathy in severe cases. The hypertension and DIC cause renal damage and the appearance of proteinuria.

> PIH is the oonnonest cause for admission to hospital during the third trimester.

PIH occurs most commonly among the following patient groups:

- primigravidae
- increased maternal age
- gross obesity
- PIH complicating an earlier pregnancy (1 in 3 chance of recurrence)
- pre-existing essential hypertension
- multiple pregnancy
- diabetes
- severe rhesus iso-immunization
- hydatidiform mole.

Signs of possible development of PIH include:

(1) an increase in diastolic blood pressure of more than 20 mmHg but still below 90 diastolic;

(2) persistent weight gain of more than 1 kg per week over any 4-week interval;

(3) oedema not only of the ankles, but also of the fingers and face, especially if still present on waking in the morning;

(4) proteinuria.

For these patients, Doppler studies of uterine blood flow would *detect a potential problem*. It may be that for these patients, as well as for those in the PIH-susceptible group above, that low-dose aspirin will be indicated. (Aspirin reduces platelet aggregation factors and may prevent DIC.)

The diagnosis of PIH is based upon:

(1) any persistently raised blood pressure of 140/90 or above after 20 weeks, but more usually after 30 weeks; (PIH does not occur before the 20th week, except in cases of hydatidiform mole.)

(2) excessive weight gain;

(3) oedema which is a normal feature of pregnancy unless severe;

(4) proteinuria.

The management of PIH will depend upon its severity. It is, therefore, important to be aware of a working method of classification:

Mild PIH	Diastolic blood pressure 90–100
Moderate PIH	Diastolic blood pressure 100–110
Severe PIH	Diastolic blood pressure > than 110 or > 90 but complicated by proteinuria

Mild PIH

When the diastolic blood pressure is found to be 90–100 mmHg, serial blood pressure readings should be made while the patient is in a resting state. (Remember to use a large blood pressure cuff on the obese patient.) If an antenatal assessment area is available, a series of accurate measurements using a Dynamap can be carried out over the course of a few hours. If the blood pressure is completely normal (below 90) for *every* recording, she should be allowed to go home and bave further blood pressure checks carried out by the community midwife. As long as these further checks are normal, she should attend the antenatal clinic again the following week. If a day assessment area is not available, then assessment as an in-patient over 24 hours is the only alternative.

Be wary of the plea, 'I always get upset when I come to the clinic'. An anxiety state does not raise the diastolic blood pressure, only the mystolic.

It is negligent to ignore the early signs of PIH.

When the diastolic blood pressure remains between 90 and 100, the patient cannot be effectively managed as an out-patient until the blood pressure is controlled.

The basis of general in-patient care will involve:

(1) rest (but not confined to bed);

(2) 4-hourly blood pressure recordings;

(3) urinalysis for proteinuria;

(4) daily or alternate day cardiotocography;

(5) kick chart;

(6) fortnightly ultrasound assessment of fetal growth;

(7) Doppler blood flow studies to detect placental dysfunction;

(8) weekly measurement of: (a) urate
                                               (b) platelets.

Hypotensive therapy may be considered necessary, as it will only be when the diastolic blood pressure can be maintained below 90 that there will be any prospect of discharging the patient home. [Hypotensive therapy is the same as for essential hypotension; p. 79] She is followed up in the antenatal clinic, with interim blood pressure checks being carried out by the community midwife. Rest should be encouraged. Until recently it was thought that lying on the left side increased placental perfusion, but this has not been borne out by Doppler studies. She should, however, be advised to avoid lying on her back so as to prevent supine hypotension.

As in essential hypertension, there is no place for diuretics which only reduce placental perfusion further.

If the blood pressure is controlled, the aim should be to deliver between 38 weeks and term.

Moderate and severe PIH

The in-patient management of this group of patients is the same as for the mild PIH group, with the exception that bed rest means *complete bed rest*.

When the early third trimester is complicated by moderate or severe PIH, hypotensive therapy becomes very important. Hypotensives do *not* influence the disease process, but may buy time for the baby if very premature, and will certainly reduce maternal risk.

> It must be remembered that delivery is the ultimate treatment for severe PIH.

When fetal maturity is satisfactory, there is no difficulty in coming to the decision to deliver. However, in the early weeks of the third trimester, the decision as to when to deliver is not so easy. The increasing risk of an intrauterine death by delaying delivery must be balanced against the risk of a neonatal death from gross prematurity.

Indications to deliver regardless of maturity:

(1) signs of severe intrauterine growth retardation, both clinically and on ultrasound/Doppler flow;

(2) diastolic blood pressure >110 despite treatment;

(3) increasing proteinuria (24-hour urinary protein);

(4) increasing urate levels;

(5) signs of imminent eclampsia;

(6) eclampsia.

As with severe essential hypertension, the decision as to the method of delivery will be based upon the degree of prematurity, the presence of complicating factors, and the favourability of the cervix. When the baby is both premature and growth-retarded, an elective Caesarean section will be the least stressful method of delivery. If an epidural is being considered, coagulation studies must first be undertaken because of the possibility of a coagulopathy.

(Imminent eclampsia and eclampsia are discussed in the chapter on antenatal emergencies.)

Intrauterine growth retardation (IUGR)

Intrauterine growth-retardation is a major cause of perinatal death. Awareness of the possibility of IUGR developing is probably the most important aspect in its detection. It must be remembered that in a significant number of cases of IUGR there is no apparent explanation.

IUGR should be anticipated in the following patient groups:

- hypertension (essential and PIH)
- antepartum haemorrhage
- multiple pregnancy
- cigarette smoking during pregnancy
- elderly primigravidae
- a previous small-for-dates baby
- a previous unexplained intrauterine death
- infection: cytomegalovirus
            malaria
            chronic urinary tract infection
            syphilis.

It is essential that patients in the above 'at risk' groups are referred early for assessment and ultrasound dating. Two biparietal diameter (BPD) measurements 4 weeks apart should resolve any dating problem or a dates/size discrepancy by the 18th week. Ultrasound dating in the late third trimester is highly inaccurate. An avoidable situation familiar to most obstetricians, is to be asked to see a patient for the first time at ?36 weeks by very uncertain dates with a query by the GP or midwife regarding fetal size and a request for ultrasound dating.

Detection of IUGR will be based upon:

(1) clinical assessment of uterine size;

(2) serial ultrasonography;

(3) serial Doppler flow studies;

(4) antenatal assessment of fetal well-being by:
    cardiotocography
    kick chart.

Clinical assessment of uterine size

The time-honoured method of assessing fetal size has been by palpation and measuring the symphysial–fundal height of the uterus. But there can be so many variables, such as an obese abdominal wall, tense abdominal muscles, and a full bladder, that the true size of the baby may be masked. However, if the examination is performed skilfully by the same observer at each antenatal visit, a reduction in the expected rate of growth may be detected. It is also often possible to detect clinically a marked reduction in the liquor volume which must then indicate a need for further investigation. Linked to the clinical assessment will be the opportunity to assess maternal weight gain. A woman who fails to gain weight in pregnancy need not necessarily be a candidate for placental insufficiency. Diet or gastrointestinal upset could account for poor or absent weight gain. However, if she is in the 'at risk' group, the poor weight gain may be significant.

Serial ultrasonography

Ultrasonography will detect a number of causes of IUGR which are associated with fetal abnormality, such as oligohydramnios resulting from renal agenesis. Ultrasound is the chief method used for detecting IUGR in the UK. Reliance upon the BPD alone will give a false sense of security. After the 28th week the BPD will become unreliable owing to the frequently-seen normal variation in head shape. Associated with intrauterine starvation, there is a loss of glycogen deposited in the liver, which is revealed by a reduction in abdominal circumference. In IUGR the head circumference and femur length will be consistent with the gestational age of the fetus, but the abdominal circumference will be small for the gestational age. The ratio of head circumference to abdominal wall circumference will therefore increase.

The liquor pool provides a valuable additional index in IUGR. A reduction in liquor volume implies poor placental function. Using an ultrasound transducer, a direct A–P representative liquor column is chosen for measurement. A liquor column measuring less than 3 cm is diagnostic of oligohydramnios. A column measuring less than 2 cm indicates severe oligohydramnios.

Serial Doppler flow studies

Doppler studies of uterine artery blood flow will be representative of placental blood flow. In a normal pregnancy, the uterine and placental circulation provide low resistance to blood flow. Therefore, blood velocity will be high during both systole and diastole. A good end-diastolic flow will confirm that there is no placental dysfunction.

The combination of serial ultrasound fetal growth monitoring and Doppler blood flow studies will permit the most accurate assessment of intrauterine growth. An increasing head circumference:abdominal circumference ratio and a significantly reduced or absent end-diastolic flow at Doppler assessment, will indicate a most serious, if not terminal, impairment of placental function.

Antenatal assessment of fetal well-being

The antenatal cardiotocograph (CTG) and kick charts have already been discussed (pp. 29–32). The poorly nourished baby will generally exhibit reduced activity. The kick chart may be the first indication of a serious problem. It must be remembered that a CTG trace will only give information regarding fetal well-being at the time that the tracing was carried out.

Many of the patients in the 'at risk' group may already be in-patients because of an associated problem, such as hypertension. The diagnosis of worsening IUGR demands admission and intensive monitoring, to include daily cardiotocography. The decision as to when to intervene and deliver the baby will depend upon the balance of risk. Will the baby have a greater chance of survival outside the uterus? When there are additional signs of intrauterine anoxia on the antenatal CTG, delivery is urgent regardless of the gestational age, if an intrauterine death is to be avoided. In this situation, delivery by elective Caesarean section will be less stressful to the baby. These babies have little in reserve to withstand asphyxia and metabolic acidosis.

Diabetes in pregnancy

> Pregnancy is a diabetogenic state. As a result, existing diabetes is aggravated by pregnancy and impaired glucose tolerance may come to light.

It is estimated that less than 1 per cent of women will have diabetes during their reproductive years. An additional 2 per cent develop gestational diabetes in pregnancy, although as many as 15 per cent of women will exhibit glycosuria in pregnancy.

Diabetes does not confer any favours upon pregnancy. Overall, the perinatal mortality rate can be as high as 50–100 per 1000 births.

As most diabetics are known to their GPs before pregnancy occurs, an important aim of antenatal care is the early detection of patients with impaired glucose tolerance who will become gestational diabetics. Although the fetal abnormality rate is not increased in gestational diabetes, detection and control is still very important, as big babies and all the other complications given above can still occur.

Effects of diabetes upon pregnancy:

- large baby (macrosomia)
  (In poorly controlled diabetes, a raised glucose level stimulates fetal pancreatic beta cells to produce insulin, leading to fat deposition in the fetus.)
- late intrauterine death
  (When control is poor, maternal ketosis may lead to fatal fetal acidosis.)
- raised fetal abnormality
  (7 per cent among insulin-dependent diabetics)
- polyhydramnios
  (This complicates up to 30 per cent of diabetic pregnancies. Hydramnios in turn may lead to an unstable lie and premature rupture of membranes.)
- pregnancy-induced hypertension
  (The incidence of PIH is three times higher than in non-diabetics. This complication increases the perinatal mortality rate.)
- bacteriuria
  (This is twice as common as among non-diabetics.)
- candida infections
- shoulder dystocia
- neonatal hypoglycaemia and respiratory distress syndrome.

Detection of gestational diabetes

Particular groups of pregnant women should be screened for gestational diabetes by carrying out a glucose tolerance test.

Indications for glucose tolerance testing:

(1) family history of diabetes in a close relative;
(2) previous big baby > 4.5 kg (10 lbs);
(3) previous unexplained stillbirth;
(4) obesity (> 85 kg);
(5) previous congenital abnormality;
(6) previous pregnancy complicated by gestational diabetes;
(7) polyhydramnios;
(8) glycosuria on two or more occasions.

Because of the poor pick-up of gestational diabetes from the presence of glycosuria, centres are increasingly turning to assessing random blood glucose levels at booking and at 28–32 weeks.

The random blood glucose levels that would indicate a glucose tolerance test are:

> > 6.1 mmol/l within 2 hours of a meal

> > 5.6 mmol/l more than 2 hours after the last meal

The diagnosis of diabetes and impaired glucose tolerance is based upon the 75 g glucose tolerance test (GTT). (See Fig. 3.1) [The glucose used for the GTT often causes nausea. 375 ml of 'Lucozade' is equivalent to 75 g glucose and is more palatable.]

Results of 75 g glucose tolerance test

Non-diabetic
- fasting blood glucose < 8 mmol/l
- 2 hour blood glucose < 8 mmol/l

Impaired glucose tolerance (gestational diabetes)
- fasting blood glucose < 8 mmol/l
- 2-hour blood glucose between 8 and 11 mmol/l

Diabetes
- fasting blood glucose > 8 mmol/l
- 2-hour blood glucose > 11 mmol/l

Insulin-dependent diabetes

The major factor in the management of diabetes in pregnancy is good control.

For the known insulin-dependent diabetic, control begins *before* pregnancy, ideally via a pre-conception clinic. Diabetics have an unusually high level of glycosylated haemoglobin (Hb A^{Ic}) in their red cells. As Hb A^{Ic} only undergoes very slow change over the course of several weeks, it is a useful indicator of overall blood glucose levels in the previous 1–3 months. Levels of Hb A^{Ic} greater than 10 per cent indicate poor control. If the Hb A^{Ic} level can be maintained below 10 per cent before pregnancy, it is more likely to be well-controlled during organogenesis with a reduction in fetal abnormality rates.

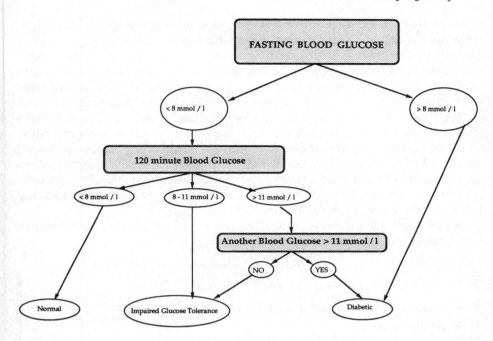

Fig. 3.1   Interpretation of a 75 g glucose tolerance test.

When pregnancy is diagnosed, early referral to the consultant unit is essential. Ideally, the pregnant diabetic should be seen in a combined antenatal/diabetic clinic attended by an obstetrician, a physician with an interest in the pregnant diabetic, and a dietician. Eventually there will also be involvement of the neo-natal paediatrician.

The woman's diet should be adjusted to 150–250 g carbohydrate per day and the weight gain maintained below 12 kg between the 20th week and delivery. She should receive three meals each day with three snacks between these, the last being just before sleeping.

In pregnancy the insulin requirements will increase. The most usual insulin regimen is to administer twice daily a short-acting soluble (Actrapid) and medium-acting isophane (Insulatard). There is thought to be some advantage to using human insulins. Good control means that the fasting blood glucose levels are kept below 5 mmol/l and random blood glucose below 6 mmol/l. If the morning fasting blood glucose level is above 6 mmol/l, the risk of increasing the evening dosage is hypoglycaemia at night. It is preferable to divide the evening dosage so that the Actrapid is used before the evening meal, and the Insulatard before retiring. The consequences of good control are a major reduction in fetal abnormality, in large babies, and in the perinatal mortality rate.

The woman is taught how to monitor her pre- and post-prandial blood glucose levels, usually by means of a blood-testing strip such as BM Stix and a reflectance meter. Urine glucose levels are of less value in monitoring the degree of control. (For the less well-motivated patient, reasonable control can be achieved by urine testing for glucose and ketones as long as there is a contact telephone number for her to use if control seems to be lost. These patients would also need to have their blood glucose levels assessed regularly in the antenatal clinic.) An overview of control is obtained by carrying out a 4-weekly Hb A^{IC} measurement.

The insulin-dependent diabetic requires full hospital antenatal care. Initially this is on a 2-weekly basis until 28 weeks, and thereafter she is seen every week.

Early ultrasonography is important so that accurate dating can be established beyond doubt. A detailed anomaly scan will exclude congenital abnormalities (neural tube defects and congenital heart disease are the commonest abnormalities in diabetic pregnancies). Serial ultrasound scans are performed to assess fetal growth and to look for polyhydramnios.

A kick chart and antenatal cardiotocography provide essential monitoring of fetal well-being.

Indications for antenatal admission

- evidence of poor diabetic control: Hb A^{IC} > 10 per cent
- polyhydramnios
- pregnancy-induced hypertension
- infection
- for in-patient fetal monitoring after 36 weeks.

If premature labour occurs, sympathomimetics such as ritodrine (Yutopar) given in an attempt to stop labour, may dramatically increase insulin requirements.

In view of the risk of sudden stillbirth, delivery is planned between 38 weeks and term. Overall, 50 per cent of diabetics are delivered by Caesarean section, but this high figure is partly due to repeat operations in multigravidae.

Indications for elective caesarean section

- a large baby
- ? disproportion
- pregnancy-induced hypertension
- malpresentation
- multiple pregnancy
- previous Caesarean section
- elderly primigravidae.

Any obstetric complication is an indication for an elective Caesarean section.

If an elective Caesarean section is performed, it is preferable if this is carried out under epidural anaesthesia, as there will be a quicker return to normal diet.

If there are absolutely no contraindications, a vaginal delivery can be contemplated. The methods used for induction are as for non-diabetic patients.

On the morning of induction, the woman should have a light breakfast and her normal dosage of short-acting insulin. A 500 ml 5 per cent dextrose infusion is set up and given 4-hourly. Soluble insulin (50 units Actrapid in 50 ml normal saline) is administered by pump (1 ml per hour = 1 unit per hour) at a rate of 1–2 units per hour titrated against hourly blood glucose levels. The aim is to maintain blood glucose levels on BM Stix at 4–5.5 mmol/l.

BM Stix	Units/hour
1	0
2	0
4.5	1
6.5	1.5
9.0	2
11.0	2.5
>17.0	3+
	(Check blood glucose)

Continuous fetal heart rate monitoring by CTG is essential.

Any worries concerning fetal well-being, or unsatisfactory progress in labour, are indications for Caesarean section.

The paediatrician must be present at delivery. The baby is closely observed on the neonatal unit for hypoglycaemia, hyperbilirubinaemia, hypocalcaemia, and respiratory distress syndrome.

Postnatally, the insulin dosage is returned to pre-pregnancy levels.

The dextrose infusion is continued until the next main meal.

It is important to discuss contraception. The combined oral contraceptive Pill is not contraindicated, although recurrent candida infections can be a problem. Once the family is complete, sterilization may be the better option.

Diabetics controlled on oral hypoglycaemic drugs

Hypoglycaemic drugs can cross the placenta and cause fetal hyperinsulinaemia. These patients should have their oral drugs changed to soluble insulin and be managed like the insulin-dependent diabetic.

Gestational diabetes

Once a woman is diagnosed as having this, a blood sugar series should be carried out while on her normal diet. If any blood glucose levels are above 5.5 mmol/l, dietary control is established with 150 g carbohydrate diet. The blood sugar series is repeated. Any further blood glucose above 5.5 mmol/l is an indication for insulin control.

Delivery is planned for between 38 weeks and term. Large babies and shoulder dystocia are the major potential problems.

The insulin is stopped after delivery. Six weeks postpartum, the glucose tolerance test is repeated. Twenty per cent of gestational diabetics will develop diet-controlled diabetes later in life. It is in the best interests of the obese gestational diabetic to lose weight, in view of the considerably increased risk (70 per cent) of later developing diabetes.

Heart disease in pregnancy

Less than 1 per cent of pregnancies in the UK are complicated by heart disease. In the Report on Confidential Enquiries into Maternal Deaths in the UK (1988–90), cardiac disease was the second commonest indirect cause of maternal death (18 deaths in the triennium). The reduced incidence of rheumatic fever and the improved results of corrective cardiac surgery, means that the proportion of deaths from congenital heart disease continues to rise, amounting to 50 per cent of the cardiac deaths.

Eight of the 9 cases of congenital heart disease and 8 of the 9 cases of acquired heart disease were considered to have had substandard care. In 7 cases, the patients disregarded medical advice to avoid becoming pregnant, and in 4 cases refused the offer of termination. Compliance with medical advice during pregnancy was often poor. The need for improved pre-conception counselling is stressed, as well as early referral to a cardiologist and subsequent combined care.

In pregnancy, the normal heart must cope with dramatic haemodynamic changes. Antenatally there is a 30 per cent increase in blood volume. By the 30th week, the cardiac output increases by 40 per cent, largely due to an increased stroke volume. The workload of the heart then remains steady until labour itself when there is a further increase in cardiac output. This is due to the rapid expansion in blood volume after the second stage of labour, when up to a litre of blood from a well-contracted uterus enters the circulation. The normal heart has no difficulty in adjusting to these changes. However, in the presence of heart disease even this normal physiological increase in workload may lead to congestive cardiac failure and pulmonary oesdema.

Any factor that might threaten to increase cardiac workload must be avoided.

Factors that may increase cardiac workload include:

- excessive physical effort
- anaemia
- pregnancy-induced hypertension
- infection:
  respiratory tract
  urinary tract
  subacute bacterial endocarditis (SBE).

Mitral stenosis is the commonest form of rheumatic heart disease. The commonest congenital defects (usually operated upon in childhood) are patent ductus and the septal defects. Congenital disorders which have a right-to-left shunt as in Eisenmenger's syndrome and uncorrected Fallot's tetralogy, carry a high maternal mortality rate and present an indication for termination of pregnancy. Very rarely, cardiomyopathy complicates late pregnancy and the postpartum period.

Patients with prosthetic mitral and aortic valves are maintained permanently on warfarin because of the risk of thrombo-embolism. Although there are teratogenic risks from warfarin therapy, it is generally considered to be the most effective anticoagulant to use in this particular situation. Intravenous heparin is substituted for warfarin from 38 weeks, reversed to cover delivery and recommenced immediately postpartum.

Most patients with heart disease will be known to their GPs. All should seek pre-pregnancy counselling. Those with right-to-left shunts such as Eisenmenger's syndrome should be advised to avoid pregnancy. Patients who are incapacitated by dyspnoea and fatigue at rest or on minimal effort, should defer plans for a pregnancy until after cardiac surgery.

The aim of antenatal care, for heart disease patients, is to prevent heart failure.

Antenatal management of cardiac patients *must* be carried out jointly by the obstetrician and cardiologist. At each attendance she is specifically questioned about dyspnoea and orthopnoea. If there is any dyspnoea, the chest is auscultated for basal rales.

Increasing dyspnoea = admission

All cardiac patients *must* have direct access to the consultant unit in the event of dyspnoea or undue fatigue.

Key points in the antenatal management of cardiac patients include:

- stop smoking
- correct anaemia
- avoid dental sepsis
- antibiotic cover for any operative procedure (tooth extraction, etc.)
- treat all infections seriously with antibiotics to avoid SBE
- adequate extra rest
- admission for problems.

If there are any signs of heart failure, the patient will require in-patient care for the duration of the pregnancy. Very occasionally there may be an indication to consider mitral valvotomy during the pregnancy.

Unless there is an obstetric contraindication, a vaginal delivery should be planned.

The key points in the management of labour in cardiac patients

- antibiotic cover
- maternal tachycardia = digitalization
- adequate analgesia:
  - epidurals are safe but avoid supine hypotension
  - morphine 15 mg intramuscularly is a good alternative
- look for signs of acute pulmonary oedema:
  - severe dyspnoea
  - haemoptysis
  - basal rales
- short second stage/elective forceps or ventouse
- care ++ during the third stage.

As long as there are no signs of heart failure, it is safer to give an oxytocic after delivery of the baby than to risk an uncontrolled bleed. The heart can be protected from the effects of a sudden increase in the circulating blood volume caused by a well-contracted uterus, by giving frusemide 40 mg intravenously early in the second stage. Having promoted a significant diuresis, syntocinon 10 units or ergometrine 0.25 mg may be given intravenously with safety.

The first 24 hours after delivery are the most crucial because of the overloading of the circulation. Careful observation is made for signs of pulmonary oedema.

Early mobilization is important so as to reduce the risks of thrombo-embolism. Any infection is treated vigorously. There is no contraindication to breast-feeding.

An elective Caesarean section will be safer than a prolonged, difficult and, and stressful labour.

Contraception should be discussed while still in hospital. There is a definite place for early post-puerperium sterilization.

Do not be too hasty in discharging the patient home.

Are the home conditions suitable? The assistance of the medical social worker can be very valuable.

Thyroid disease in pregnancy

Hyperthyroidism

Hyperthyroidism occurs in one in 500 pregnancies. The majority of thyrotoxic women are already on treatment for their hyperthyroidism pre-pregnancy.

In a normal pregnancy, the free thyroxine (T_4), free triiodothyronine (T_3), and thyroid-stimulating hormone (TSH) are unchanged. In thyrotoxicosis, the free T_4 and T_3 are increased and the TSH is decreased.

Carbimazole 15 mg three times daily, is the drug of choice. The aim is to keep free T_4 in the high normal range. Carbimazole crosses the placenta, and excessive dosage suppresses fetal TSH, resulting in hypothyroidism and goitre. To avoid this, carbimazole should be stopped at 37 weeks and is recommenced postnatally. As carbimazole appears in breast milk, these babies should not be breast-fed.

Propylthiouracil may be a better alternative to carbimazole, and may be safe for the fetus as it does not cross the placental barrier so readily.

Maternal tachycardia is treated with propranolol.

The main antenatal risk of failing to treat thyrotoxicosis adequately is premature labour. Regardless of whether or not maternal thyrotoxicosis is being treated, congenital thyrotoxicosis can affect 10 per cent of babies, due to maternal thyroid-stimulating antibodies crossing the placenta. These babies can be detected if the level of long-acting thyroid stimulator protector (LATS/P) antibody in maternal blood is above 20 U/ml after the 30th week of pregnancy.

The appearance of congenital thyrotoxicosis can be delayed for up to 10 days, when restlessness, tachycardia, and feeding problems become apparent. Treatment is with carbimazole and propranolol.

Hypothyroidism

One in a 100 patients will have hypothyroidism. These women are usually on treatment before pregnancy as the condition commonly causes anovulatory infertility. The pre-pregnancy thyroxine dosage may need to be increased once the woman is pregnant, as the dosage is weight-related. The aim of treatment is to keep the patient euthyroid. Thyroxine 2 μg/kg body weight daily should achieve this.

Untreated hypothyroidism increases the risk of abortion, premature labour, intrauterine death, and fetal abnormality.

Rhesus iso-immunization

In Caucasian communities, 15 per cent of the population will be rhesus-negative. As 75 per cent of rhesus-negative women will have a rhesus-positive baby, this is the major cause of rhesus iso-immunization.

> It is a normal event for fetal blood cells to cross the placenta and enter the maternal circulation.

If the fetal blood group is incompatible with the maternal ABO group, any fetal cells will be destroyed by maternal anti-A and anti-B before there is time for iso-immunization to occur.

If *sufficient* fetal cells of an ABO-compatible group are transfused into the maternal circulation, they will *not* be destroyed by the maternal immunological system. In the majority of cases (the response is variable), the rhesus antigen will stimulate antibody formation. The resulting antibodies are both the large macroimmunoglobulin IgM which cannot pass across the placenta, and the smaller IgG immunoglobulin which can cross the placenta and enter the fetal circulation.

> It is extremely rare for antibody formation to develop in time to affect the first pregnancy.

The IgM antibody develops 7 days after stimulation, whereas the IgG antibody only appears after 21 days. It is for this reason that a first pregnancy is unlikely to be affected, as the major stimulation occurs at delivery. However, it will only require a small feto-maternal transfusion of rhesus-positive cells in a subsequent pregnancy to stimulate a vigorous antibody response. The IgG antibodies will cross the placenta and haemolyse fetal red cells, causing haemolytic disease.

Haemolytic disease of the fetus may take the form of **congenital haemolytic anaemia** or **hydrops fetalis**. Hyarops fetalis results from fetal cardiac failure and ascites due to the severity of the anaemia and hypoxia. After delivery, the bilirubin resulting from fetal red cell haemolysis is no longer removed by the maternal circulation. The fetal liver is unable to cope, leading to increasing jaundice known as **icterus gravis neonatorum**. If the levels of bilirubin rise above 350 μmol/litre, this can damage the basal ganglia of the brain and cause **kernicterus**.

Management of rhesus-negative pregnancy without antibodies

Rhesus iso-inmunization is largely preventable.

If any complication arises which may lead to a feto-maternal transfusion, the unsensitized rhesus-negative woman must be protected with anti-D immuno-globulin.

Feto-maternal transfusion may occur during:

- abortion (threatened → complete)
             (therapeutic abortion)
- ectopic pregnancy
- amniocentesis
- external cephalic version
- antepartum haemorrhage
- delivery (vaginal or Caesarean section).

If any potential immunizing factor occurs before the 20th week, anti-D immunoglobulin 50 μg (250 IU) is given by intramuscular injection within 48–72 hours of the incident. After the 20th week the anti-D immunoglobulin dosage is doubled.

The presence of rhesus antibodies is assessed antenatally at booking, 28 weeks, and 36 weeks by indirect Coombs' testing or direct quantitative analysis.

After delivery of the placenta, a cord blood sample is taken for fetal blood group and rhesus group, haemoglobin, bilirubin, and direct Coombs' test.

A maternal blood sample is taken for rhesus antibodies and for a Kleihauer test to determine the quantity of fetal cells present per low-power field using an acid elution technique (50 cells per 50 low-power fields is equivalent to a feto-maternal transfusion of 5 ml).

If the baby is rhesus-positive and there are no rhesus antibodies present, ALL rhesus-negative women are given anti-D immunoglobulin 100 μg (500 IU) intramuscularly within 48–72 hours of delivery. This is increased if the feto-maternal bleed is large (20 μg will be required for every ml of fetal blood). If there are indications of a large feto-maternal bleed, it is worth while to carry out an indirect Coombs' test 24 hours after the anti-D has been given. If negative, indicating that no antibody is present, the Kleihauer test is repeated. Additional anti-D may be required.

> Anti-D is not given if the baby is rhesus-negative or if maternal rhesus antibodies are present.

Management of rhesus-negative pregnancy with antibodies

Once rhesus antibodies are detected, the paternal blood group and genotype should be assessed, as if he is heterozygous rhesus-positive, there is a 50 per cent chance of the baby being rhesus-negative.

Maternal antibody screening must be repeated every 2–4 weeks. The level of circulating maternal anti-D is a poor indicator of the severity of the disease process. Indeed, the antibody titre will rise in pregnancy, even if the fetus in the current pregnancy is rhesus-negative.

> If the antibody titre reaches 5 IU or higher, and especially if it is rising rapidly, referral to a specialist centre for cordocentesis is a matter of some urgency.

In the first affected pregnancy, the centre may initially only carry out ultrasound surveillance and defer cordocentesis until 28 weeks. Ultrasonography is very important in such cases so as to detect the early presence of fetal ascites and even scalp oedema. Hydropic changes are no longer associated with an invariably fatal outcome. If a high antibody titre is found at early booking or if there has been a previous seriously affected pregnancy, the cordocentesis can be brought forwards to as early as 18 weeks. Cordocentesis will permit determination of the fetal haemoglobin and haematocrit so that the degree of fetal red cell haemolysis can be accurately assessed. This can be repeated at regular intervals.

Before the availability of cordocentesis, the only way of attempting to determine the severity of the rhesus iso-immunization was by amniocentesis. The degree of fetal red cell haemolysis correlated reasonably well with the level of bilirubin in the amniotic fluid. By means of spectrophotometry, the optical density of the liquor was assessed and plotted onto a Liley graph. The Liley graph zones were used as a guide to assess the severity of the iso-immunization. However, the severity of fetal anaemia cannot always be accurately determined by means of optical density.

In an affected pregnancy, treatment will be determined by fetal maturity and the severity of the disease process.

It is maturity that will determine the timing of delivery.

In severe rhesus disease, the fetus will die *in utero* or, if labour is induced, will be unable to survive after delivery because of gross prematurity. Therefore, the aim of treatment is to 'buy time and maturity' for as long as safety will permit.

Treatment options in severe disease include:

(1) **intrauterine transfusion** every 2 weeks between 18 and 32 weeks using ultrasound-directed cordocentesis;

(2) **plasmaphoresis** to reduce extremely high maternal antibody levels is now infrequently performed owing to the improved ultrasound guided techniques of intrauterine transfusion;

(3) **premature induction**.

During intrauterine transfusion, it is essential to avoid overloading the fetal circulation. Three-quarters of the required blood is transfused directly into the cord and the remaining quarter is instilled into the fetal peritoneal cavity. The overall fetal mortality rate resulting directly from intrauterine transfusion is 10 per cent.

If the fetus is thought to be only mildly affected, labour is induced at 38 weeks. The more severely affected fetus may require earlier delivery. As these patients are multiparous, there is usually no difficulty in inducing labour. Continuous CTG monitoring is essential. If delivery is indicated before 34 weeks, an elective Caesarean section is likely to be the least traumatic delivery for the baby. Remember that the baby may still have to cope with an exchange transfusion.

After delivery, the baby is assessed to determine the effects of the haemolytic disease. The severity of the disease will be shown by the degree of anaemia, bilirubin level, and a positive Coombs' test.

If the haemoglobin is above 14.8 g/dl, the baby is only mildly affected. Mild jaundice may develop which will respond to phototherapy.

Severely affected babies will require exchange transfusion with cross-matched, rhesus-negative blood (which cannot be haemolysed by circulating antibodies). Repeated transfusions are often necessary. These will restore the haemoglobin to normal and reduce the bilirubin and antibody levels.

In theory it should be possible to completely prevent rhesus disease. But there will always be some rhesus-negative women who will abort at home, and either not realize it or fail to inform their GPs. As a result, they will not receive anti-D immunoglobulin. Sadly, there are still cases of women who do not receive anti-D, in spite of aborting in hospital, because the blood group was not screened and it was simply 'forgotten'.

For some women who have had a disastrous history of recurrent pregnancy loss, there may be a place for donor insemination using sperm from a rhesus-negative donor.

It would be ideal if all rhesus-negative women with a rhesus-positive partner received anti-D immunoglobulin at 28 and 34 weeks. However, this would have major implications upon the available supply of anti-D and will need to wait until monoclonal anti-D can be produced in quantity. With further reduction in the incidence of rhesus iso-immunization, the rarer antibody problems, such as anti-Kell and anti-Duffy, will become relatively more common than rhesus antibodies.

Cephalo-pelvic disproportion (CPD)

Disproportion exists when there is a significant reduction in one or more of the major diameters of the pelvis. The pelvis may not always be of the correct proportion either in shape or in size. In practice, the important relationship is between the size and position of the fetal head and the size and shape of the pelvis.

> A malpresentation of a *normal-sized fetal head* may lead to disproportion even if the pelvis is of *normal size and shape*.

Cephalo-pelvic disproportion (CPD) will occur when the fetal head is too large for the pelvis.

CPD-will affect less than 2 per cent of the obstetric population of the UK. The improvement in nutrition and community health has made rickets and osteomalacia conditions of the past. Bone diseases such as osteomyelitis and TB and the exotic congenital pelvic malformations are rarely seen. However, spinal conditions such as spondylolithesis may cause CPD.

Factors associated with cephalo-pelvic disproportion

- height is less than 150 cm (5 feet)
- past history of a fractured pelvis
- a previous prolonged labour
- a previous difficult forceps delivery
- a previous large baby
- a past history of shoulder dystocia
- when on palpation the fetus feels excessively large
- a high head at term in a primigravida.

Many small women will have no difficulty in delivering babies of a normal size. But babies do tend to increase in size with successive pregnancies. A woman of small stature may have had no difficulty in delivering a 3 kg baby, but CPD may occur if the next baby is 4 kg.

It must be remembered that every primigravida is an unknown quantity with regard to her future performance in labour.

There is a regrettable tendency nowadays to omit antenatal pelvic assessment of the primigravida until she presents in labour. There are problems apart from those relating to the pelvic brim that it would be advantageous to know about and plan for, such as a reduced pelvic outlet.

Clinical assessment of the pelvis should be carried out on every primigravida at 36–38 weeks, unless it is already known that she will be having an elective Caesarean section.

The pelvic assessment should be carried out by an experienced obstetrician. (The details of the information to be gained from such an assessment have been given on p. 26.)

It is worth restating that the best pelvimeter of the pelvic inlet is the fetal head. An engaged head is proof that there is no disproportion at the pelvic brim. The diagnosis of 'engagement' should be made on a combination of abdominal palpation and vaginal examination.

Disproportion need not only arise at the pelvic brim. The pelvic assessment may have revealed a reduced outlet with a narrow sub-pubic angle. This may be of a sufficient degree to make an entry on the notes suggesting that a 'trial of forceps' should be carried out in theatre if there is delay in the second stage of labour

If there is any doubt about the capacity of the pelvis, a CAT scan pelvimetry or an erect lateral X-ray pelvimetry is indicated.

> ALWAYS look at the film. DON'T simply rely upon the measurements given on a report.

If there is thought to be borderline brim disproportion only, *and no other obstetric problem*, a 'trial of labour' can be planned (see p. 191). In other words, if the fetal head can negotiate the pelvic brim, there should be no further problems.

The plan of management should be thoroughly explained to the woman. She must fully appreciate that in the event of progress in labour being poor, a Caesarean section will be carried out.

> Cephalo-pelvic disproportion must be understood to only refer to a cephalic presentation. Any doubts about pelvic capacity in a breech presentation will ALWAYS indicate a need for Caesarean section.

High head at term in the primigravida

> In 10 per cent of primigravidae, engagement of the fetal head will only occur in labour.

In the majority of primigravid pregnancies, the fetal head will engage by the 37th week. Obstetricians are frequently asked by GPs to urgently assess the problem of the primigravida with a non-engaged high head at term. The concern and urgency are due to the possibility that there may be either a placenta praevia or cephalo-pelvic disproportion. These two conditions, while not the commonest causes of a high head, are potentially the most serious.

The commonest cause of a high head at term in a primigravida is an occipito-posterior position of the head.

The main causes of a high head at term in a primigravida include:

- occipito-posterior position and deflexed head
- wrong dates (36 weeks instead of term)
- full bladder or bowel
- pendulous abdomen
- polyhydramnios
- hydrocephaly leading to cephalo-pelvic disproportion
- an already engaged undiagnosed twin(!)
- malpresentation such as brow presentation
- placenta praevia
- true disproportion where the pelvis is clinically small
- pelvic tumours (ovarian cyst or fibroid)
- among Afro-Caribbean women the pelvis tends to be very shallow and with a high angle of inclination at the pelvic brim; the head may still be palpable abdominally when engaged on vaginal examination.

These patients require a skilled pelvic examination, but not until placenta praevia has been excluded by ultrasonography. The presence of pelvic tumours can be excluded by examination, although it is unlikely that these will have been missed by ultrasound.

Abnormal presentations in the antenatal clinic

The antenatal management only of abnormal presentations is discussed in this section. Their management in labour is discussed later.

The abnormal presentations that can be detected antenatally are:

- breech presentation
- unstable lie.

Breech presentation

At 30 weeks' gestation, 20 per cent of pregnancies present as a breech. At full term this number is reduced to 3 per cent.

> The major causes of breech presentation include:
>
> - prematurity
> - extended legs splinting the fetal trunk
> - uterine septum 'fixing' the fetus
> - hydrocephaly
> - twin pregnancy.

Antenatal care of a breech presentation during the third trimester is normal, apart from the decision as to whether or not to carry out external cephalic version (ECV). The argument against ECV is that those babies that can be turned are the ones that will undergo spontaneous version anyway. Also, ECV is not free of risk. (See Table 3.2)

Probably the majority of obstetricians in the UK will *gently* attempt ECV at 32–34 weeks unless there is a contraindication to do so.

> Contraindications to ECV include:
>
> - major threat to abort earlier in the pregnancy
> - antepartum haemorrhage
> - previous Caesarean section scar
> - any complicating factor, e.g. elderly primigravida; hypertension
> - when a Caesarean section is going to be performed regardless of the presentation

It is essential to check the rhesus group of the woman before carrying out ECV. The rhesus-negative patient must have blood taken before and after the attempted procedure for Kleihauer testing and rhesus antibodies. Anti-D immunoglobulin is administered on a routine basis. No force is applied to encourage the fetus to undergo a somersaulting manoeuvre. ECV should never be carried out under sedation or general anaesthesia. In such situations, the woman is unable to protest (even by frowning!) and it is difficult to resist applying just a little bit more force than is safe. When an ECV has been successfully performed, it is important to listen to the fetal heart afterwards to ensure that there is no bradycardia. If there is a bradycardia, the problem may be a short cord which has been put under tension. The fetus should be turned back into

Table 3.2 Risks and advantages of attempting ECV

Risks of attempting ECV	Advantages resulting from ECV

Abruptio placentae
Fetal distress
Premature labour
Rhesus iso-immunization in the
  rhesus-negative patient
Cord entanglement which may come
  under pressure or tension during
  descent in labour
	Perinatal mortality for cephalic
	presentations is one-teeth of that for
	breeches
	If cephalic, there is a greater chance
	of a successful vaginal delivery; a
	persistent breech for many patients
	will be an indication for elective
	Caesarean section

the breech position in a reverse manoeuvre. A check for vaginal bleeding is also made. If the ECV has been trouble-free, as is usually the case, the patient should attend the antenatal clinic again the following week, so that the presentation can be reassessed. Unless the uterus is very lax or over-distended, once in a cephalic presentation, the fetus will tend to remain in that position.

In the event of the presentation remaining breech, it will be necessary to make a decision as to the method of delivery. There are only two options, vaginal breech delivery or elective Caesarean section.

The cardinal rule relating to the management of a breech pregnancy is:

A breech presentation + any complication = Caesarean section

Contraindications to vaginal delivery

(1) big baby (perinatal mortality increases with birth weight above 3.3 kg, regardless of how many successful vaginal deliveries she has had in the past);

(2) poor obstetric history (such as previous stillbirth);

(3) previous Caesarean section and no subsequent vaginal delivery (there is no place for a trial of scar);

(4) evidence of a seduced pelvis (the verdict of a trial of labour for borderline brim disproportion comes too late, when the baby is delivered up to the neck);

(5) hypertension;

(6) elderly primigravidae;

(7) diabetes;

(8) footling breech presentation (increased risk of cord prolapse).

Conditions to be fulfilled before deciding upon vaginal breech delivery

- there is absolutely no evidence of disproportion:
     clinical pelvic assessment;
     CAT scan pelvimetry; or
     erect lateral X-ray pelvimetry
- the baby is not clinically large (? ultrasound weight estimation)
- there is no other complication.

It is very important that the woman is fully aware of the plan of management. She must appreciate that if any problem arises in labour, even at the end of the first stage, it will still be safer to deliver by Caesarean section. (The management of breech labour is discussed in the appropriate intrapartum section.)

Unstable lie

In the majority of pregnancies, the lie of the fetus becomes stable and longitudinal in the last few weeks of pregnancy. An unstable lie exists when the lie of the fetus is constantly changing. Even in the course of the same day, the lie can be longitudinal (cephalic or breech), oblique, or transverse. This does not usually present any serious problem before the 36th week.

The factors that will contribute to an unstable lie are a large, lax, over-distended uterus, or a space-occupying mass in the pelvis or uterus which is preventing engagement of the head or breech.

The chief causes of unstable lie

(1) multiparity (poor uterine tone);
(2) polyhydramnios (an over-distended uterus provides more room to allow the fetus to adopt a lie other than longitudinal);
(3) placenta praevia;
(4) large pelvic mass (cervical fibroid or ovarian cyst impacted within the pelvis);
(5) no obvious cause to be found.

It should be noted that a persistent transverse lie (shoulder presentation) is a stable condition and will not vary from day to day. Uterine malformations such as a subseptate uterus are a possible cause of a fixed transverse lie.

When there is a malpresentation resulting from an unstable lie, there is a tendency for labour to begin by spontaneous rupture of the membranes (SROM). If the lie is other than longitudinal, there is a major risk of cord prolapse. The chance of this occuring before 36 weeks is slight, but is considerably increased after the 38th week.

If the lie has been shown to be unstable by the 36th week, ultrasonography is important, chiefly to exclude placenta praevia.

> In unstable lie, vaginal examination is deferred until placenta praevia has been excluded by ultrasonography.

A woman with an unstable lie should be admitted to hospital by 38 weeks, so that in the event of SROM and a cord prolapse, geographically she will be in the safest place. Yet even admission to hospital is no guarantee that a cord prolapse will not have fatal consequences for the baby. The woman must be instructed to *immediately* inform the nursing staff if there is any loss of fluid vaginally. Vaginal examination by trained midwifery staff must be rapidly performed so as to exclude cord prolapse.

There does not seem to be any particular benefit in carrying out daily external version to a longitudinal lie. The unstable lie will simply recur. However, the reduction in liquor volume closer to term may eventually encourage the lie to remain longitudinal. If the lie remains unstable by 42 weeks, the decision will need to be made to carry out either an elective Caesarean section or a stabilizing induction. If it is decided to induce labour, a syntocinon infusion is set up with the fetus in a longitudinal lie. When contractions commence, as long as the lie remains longitudinal, an artificial rupture of membranes (ARM) is performed in theatre with all preparations for Caesarean section standing by in the event of a cord prolapse. If labour should commence and the lie be other than longitudinal, Caesarean section is the only safe option.

Multiple pregnancy

The incidence of naturally-occuring twins is 1 in 80, triplets 1 in 8000, and quadruplets one in 800 000. There is an increased incidence in multiple pregnancies owing to ovarian hyperstimulation with gonadotrophins and to Assisted Conception programmes. Since 1st August 1991, in the UK, the Human Fertilisation and Embryology Authority (HFEA), have limited the number of eggs replaced in GIFT (gamete intra-fallopian transfer) and the number of embryos transferred in IVF (*in vitro* fertilization) to a maximum of three. When implantation techniques improve, this figure may well be reduced to two.

Twins may either be uniovular (monozygotic, monochorionic, identical) or, more commonly, binovular (dyzygotic, dichorionic, non-identical).

The possibility of a multiple pregnancy is always borne in mind when there is a history of ovulation induction, a very strong family history, and early significant hyperemesis. The majority of multiple pregnancies are diagnosed by routine ultrasound at the antenatal booking visit. But there will always be patients who have never had a scan or who only present themselves for the first time when in labour, having had no antenatal care. Rarely in such patients, a multiple pregnancy may remain undiagnosed until after the oxytocic has been given following the birth of the first baby.

Clinically a multiple pregnancy is suggested by:

- a uterus that is large for dates
- multiple fetal parts (a lot of baby!)
- more than two poles palpable (3rd trimester)
- two fetal hearts heard (two observers listening simultaneously for minute with a variation of more than 10 beats per minute in the two heart rates).

A multiple pregnancy can present numerous problems antenatally. These problems are increased for the higher order pregnancies (triplets or more).

Preterm labour is the major antenatal hazard in a multiple pregnancy.

Antenatal problems in a multiple pregnancy include:

(1) **exacerbation of all the minor pregnancy complaints:**
nausea and vomiting/hyperemesis
backache
varicose veins and haemorrhoids
constipation
abdominal discomfort
dyspnoea on effort

(2) **anaemia** (increased iron and folic acid requirements. Good diet important. Supplementary iron and folic acid from 20 weeks);

(3) **acute pyelonephritis;**

(4) PRETERM LABOUR;

(5) **pregnancy-induced hypertension;**

(6) **intrauterine growth retardation** (IUGR);

(7) **intrauterine death;**

(8) **placenta praevia** (owing to the larger placental surface area, although there is a larger uterine cavity to accommodate it);

(9) **polyhydramnios** (this can be acute in uniovular twins);

(10) **malpresentations.**

Antenatal management of multiple pregnency

Once a multiple pregnancy has been diagnosed, the patient should be advised of potential problems and the steps that can be taken to deal with them should they arise. She should be warned of the possible need for antenatal admission and should make contingency plans well in advance for the care of other children in the family.

All multiple pregnancies must be booked into a consultant unit with special care neonatal facilities. Detailed ultrasonography at 18 weeks should exclude any major fetal abnormality. Thereafter serial ultrasound scans, initially every 4 weeks, and then fortnightly after 24 weeks, is an essential part of management. IUGR and polyhydramnios may be then be detected early.

> Full hospital antenatal care is advisable after the 24th week.

Fetal movement checks (kick chart) are made after the 28th week, but 20 separate movements (as opposed to 10 for a singleton pregnancy) must be observed.

Supplementary iron and folic acid preidarations are important to prevent the otherwise likely occurence of both iron-deficiency and megaloblastic anaemias. Adequate rest from 28 weeks becomes especially important. In an uncomplicated twin pregnancy, there is no evidence that routine admission to hospital and bed rest between 28 and 32 weeks prevents premature labour. However, all patients should have ready access to admission if they find their normal day-to-day activity too tiring. It must be remembered that it is very difficult to do absolutely nothing at home as there will always be some domestic demands. To complicate matters, it is usually the case that the patient with a large and demanding family, will probably be the one who will most resist admission for rest. If admitted to hospital for rest, serial cardiotocography is valuable as an additional monitor of fetal well-being.

> All complications are treated as for a singleton pregnancy. Hypertension *always* indicates a need for admission for assessment and probable treatment.

Triplets and higher order pregnancies are more commonly seen as a result of assisted conception techniques. The perinatal mortality among such pregnancies is considerably increased because of the increased risk of preterm labour. It is quite normal for the uterus of a triplet pregnancy at 28 weeks to be equivalent in size to a full-term uterus. The tendency to go into premature labour is not surprising. Serial scans to measure the length and dilatation of the cervical canal from the 15th week can be valuable. If there is evidence of cervical shortening or dilatation, there may very occasionally be a need to consider a cervical circumsuture to give additional support to the pregnancy, but this is not helpful as a routine procedure. From 24–26 weeks, it is advisable to admit all these patients for prolonged rest in hospital. If the uterus is not particularly tense it may be possible initially to allow weekend leave to go home *to rest* and have a break from the hospital routine. However, if the uterus should be tense, or if uncomfortable contractions are experienced, there is a place for the use of sympathomimetic drugs such as ritodrine and salbutamol. In the event of a very early preterm delivery, the major hazard to the babies will be respiratory distress syndrome (RDS). From 26 weeks it is worth while to attempt to reduce the severity of RDS by giving two intramuscular injections of dexamethazone, 12 mg 12-hourly, and repeating this on a weekly basis until the end of the 33rd week. The aim in these cases is to buy time. Women who have been through procedures such as GIFT or IVF after a long infertility history, are usually highly motivated and only too happy to stay in hospital if it is going to increase the likelihood of a happy and successful outcome. From 24 weeks, fortnightly ultrasound scans are carried out to assess fetal growth. Once a triplet pregnancy reaches 34 weeks, the uterine size can be vast, causing very considerable discomfort. Labour invariably occurs spontaneously before 36 weeks. Delivery should be by elective Caesarean section. It is essential that there is close communication between obstetrician and neonatal paediatrician, as the arrival of three premature babies requiring intensive care/special care services at the same time, can have long-term implications for the resources of even the best equipped neonatal units.

> 25 per cent of twin pregnancies are complicated by premature labour before 36 weeks.

A significant proportion of twins have some degree of intrauterine growth retardation. The birth weight of each twin is, therefore, usually less than the weight of a singleton pregnancy of the same maturity. For this reason, the aim is to intervene and induce labour in uncomplicated twin pregnancies by 38 weeks.

Certain patients with a multiple pregnancy should not be permitted to labour.

> The indications for elective Caesarean section include:
>
> * elderly primigravidae
> * diabetes
> * previous Caesarean section scar 'untried' by a subsequent 'trial of scar'
> * first twin transverse lie
> * poor obstetric history
> * all triplets and other higher order pregnancies.

(For the management of twin labour see chapter on intrapartum care.)

Polyhydramnios

Polyhydramnios (or hydramnios) occurs when there is a demonstrable increase in the volume of amniotic fluid.

The liquor volume normally increases to a maximum of 1.5 litres by 38 weeks, and then diminishes towards term and beyond. The liquor is formed from fetal urine and the amnion. There is a constant circulation and turnover of amniotic fluid, with the production of urine by the fetus which is then swallowed and in part excreted via the placenta. Anything which prevents fetal swallowing or leads to an increased production of liquor by the amnion will lead to poly-hydramnios, with liquor volumes often being considerably in excess of 3 litres. Polyhydramnios will complicate 1 in 250 pregnancies.

Causes of polyhydramnios

(1) **unknown** (50 per cent of cases);

(2) **fetal abnormality** (30 per cent of cases):
   anencephaly (due to an inability to swallow liquor and a failure to produce anti-diurectic hormone)
   oesophageal atresia
   duodenal atresia
   spina bifida;

(3) **diabetes** (due to a large baby with a large placenta and increased surface area of amnion);

(4) **multiple pregnancy** (especially uniovular twins);

(5) **severe rhesus iso-immunization** (hydrops fetalis);

(6) **severe pregnancy-induced hypertension**;

(7) **chorio-angioma of the placenta** (benign tumour which produces a transudate).

The diagmosis of polyhydramnios is usually made as a result of clinical examination.

The signs of polyhydramnios

- the uterus is large for dates and tense
- fluid thrill
- ballottement of fetal parts
- muffled fetal heart sounds
- unstable lie.

Sometimes the first indication as to the development of polyhydramnios will come from routine ultrasonography. Liquor columns can increase to above 8 cm.

Polyhydramnios most commonly commences after 32 weeks and develops gradually. This 'chronic' polyhydramnios slowly increases as pregnancy progresses and produces symptoms of discomfort related to the over-distension of the uterus. It is rare for pain to be a feature of the condition. An unstable lie is common.

An acute form of polyhydramnios can develop in uniovular twins, with a sudden and dramatic increase in uterine size. The excess liquor usually only affects one amniotic cavity. Acute polyhydramnios can present as early as 20 weeks. Severe pain is the chief feature owing to the great tension affecting the abdominal wall. Other symptoms include dyspnoea and vomiting. The tense and tender uterus can mimic abruptio placentae, except for the absence of shock and bleeding. The skin of the abdomen is stretched and shiny with a glazed appearance. There is a fluid thrill present, but the uterine tension is so great that fetal parts cannot be palpated.

The major risks of polyhydramnios, whether acute or chronic, are premature labour and the problems associated with spontaneous rupture of the membranes (SROM).

Management of polyhydramnios
When polyhydramnios causes symptoms of discomfort, admission for rest becomes necessary. The patient should avoid lying flat on her back, as supine hypotensive syndrome can occur. When lying on her side, pillows beneath the abdomen give comforting support. If not already performed, detailed ultrasonography and a glucose tolerance test are carried out. In the absence of fetal abnormality, the aim of in-patient treatment is to try to prolong pregnancy and avoid premature labour. Occasionally, an amniocentesis is helpful to decompress a grossly distended and tense uterus. After placental localization, 500–1000 ml of amniotic fluid is removed, which should minimize the risk of accidentally

inducing labour. This will only give temporary benefit as liquor reforms rapidly. Repeated tappings may be required to bring about long-term relief of acute abdominal pain.

> If SROM should occur, an immediate vaginal examination is essential to exclude cord prolapse.

When a fetal abnormality is found, there is little to be gained by prolonging the pregnancy. Labour should be induced. Similarly, when abdominal pain and discomfort are severe, induction of labour may be the most appropriate treatment.

> To simply carry out an amniotomy is unwise.

Gross polyhydramnios may encourage a malpresentation which cannot be palpated because of the tenseness of the abdominal wall. Preliminary ultrasonography or even X-ray will indicate the lie of the fetus.

> The risks of amniotomy or of SROM include:
>
> - prolapsed cord
> - placental site retraction causing fetal distress
> - abruptio placentae.

The slow removal of 1–2 litres of liquor by amniocentesis will decompress the uterus and, as long as the lie is longitudinal, a fore-water rupture *in theatre* can be performed. In the event of a cord prolapse or antepartum haemorrhage, a Caesarean section can be carried out with speed. To perform the amniotomy in a delivery room, and be faced by an acute problem when the operating theatre is already in use is an avoidable nightmare! (A useful tip: wear a plastic apron and boots. This can be a damp experience for the operator!)

> Induction of labour in theatre is preferable to uncontrolled SROM and its associated problems.

As in multiple pregnancy, the uterus that has been over-distended by poly-hydramnios may not be efficient in labour. The first and second stages can be prolonged and postpartum haemorrhage can be a major complication. A syntocinon infusion can be very helpful.

> After delivery of the baby, a gastric tube must be passed so as to detect oesophageal atresia.

Oligohydramnios

> Oligohydramnios occurs when there is a demonstrable reduction in the volume of the amniotic fluid.

Clinically, the uterus is small for the expected dates. When this occurs during the second trimester it is usually linked to a fetal renal abnormality such as renal agenesis. The absence of fetal urine output dramatically reduces the total liquor volume. The diagnosis is made by ultrasound examination of the fetal kidneys and bladder. These babies do not survive.

Oligohydramnios is a feature of intrauterine growth retardation and of post-maturity. The reduction in liquor volume can be appreciated clinically, and when noted is highly significant. On ultrasonography, an A–P liquor column of 3 cm is diagnostic of oligohydramnios. The condition is severe if the liquor column is reduced to less than 2 cm. If the fetus is otherwise viable, delivery is indicated. Fetal distress in labour is a common occurrence requiring emergency operative delivery. At delivery, the baby's skin has a dry and leathery feel. Positional deformities such as talipes and wry neck may be present.

Prolonged pregnancy and postmaturity

Eighty-eight per cent of pregnancies will deliver between 38 and 42 weeks. It is interesting that less than 5 per cent of babies are actually born on the calculated expected date of delivery. Postmaturity complicates only 6 per cent of pregnancies in that they have gone beyond 42 weeks.

In the uncomplicated prolonged (but not postmature) pregnancy, no interference is necessary. If a pregnancy reaches 42 weeks, this is not a magic number that implies 'panic'! However, *if one is sure of the dates*, this landmark is generally regarded as an indication to induce labour.

The diagnosis of postmaturity will depend upon accurate knowledge of the dates and is based upon early estimation of uterine size in the first trimester and ultrasound dating before the 20th week. The placenta undergoes a rapid ageing process beyond 42 weeks. The reduction in placental efficiency and perfusion will reduce fetal oxygenation. The unstressed fetus may be able to withstand this anoxia, but the eventual onset of labour may embarrass the placental circulation, leading to sudden acute fetal distress and intrauterine death.

When there has been a major threat to abort or there has been evidence of an earlier abruption, it should be assumed that the placenta will be less efficient as term approaches. Similarly, it would be foolhardy to allow women with hypertensive disorders, diabetes, poor obstetric histories, and premium pregnancies (elderly primigravidae and significant major infertility) to become postmature.

Postmaturity should never be permitted to feature in pregnancies complicated by other problems.

Special vigilance is required once a pregnancy goes past term and is becoming prolonged. The patient should be asked to be particularly conscientious over keeping her kick chart and not hesitate to contact the hospital if she does not achieve her 10 movements within 12 hours. In that event a CTG that day is essential. If, on palpation, there is thought to be a reduction in amniotic fluid volume, urgent assessment by ultrasonography is indicated to confirm the oligohydramnios. Decelerations on an unstressed antenatal CTG or confirmation of oligohydramnios are indications for delivery. The clinical situation may indicate a need for Caesarean section rather than vaginal delivery.

Labour itself must be very closely monitored because of the risk of sudden acute fetal distress. Continuous CTG is wise. Labour tends to be prolonged with poor moulding of the harder skull bones. Finally, when the fetus has been well grown and is thought to be large, watch out for those shoulders. Shoulder dystocia can be the final nightmare of postmaturity.

4   Antenatal emergencies

Severe hyperemesis gravidarum

Severe intractable vomiting of all ingested fluids and solids is now a relatively uncommon problem in early pregnancy. Dehydration, ketosis, and weight loss are early consequences of the condition. If left untreated there is the risk of rapid deterioration. Exceedingly rarely, liver failure, jaundice, and polyneuritis can develop, until finally the continued starvation leads to encephalopathy and death in coma.

> If vomiting develops to the point of being unable to tolerate fluids, admission to hospital is essential.

In itself, admission can be very beneficial and gives support to the significance of there being psychological factors in the aetiology of hyperemesis.

Once in hospital, a history is taken and an examination is carried out. The vomiting has usually been long-standing with a number of different antiemetic preparations having already been tried, resulting in only temporary improvements. Constipation is a common feature. On examination, the woman is usually very lethargic. There may be quite marked signs of dehydration, with sunken eyes and a dry tongue. Ketosis will be evident with acetone on the breath and ketones in the urine.

> If ultrasonography has not yet been performed in the pregnancy, this is an important investigation in order to exclude hydatidiform mole. A multiple pregnancy may also be found.

Blood is taken for a full blood count, urea and electrolytes, blood sugar, liver function, and thyroid function tests. All urine passed is tested for ketones, sugar, protein, and bile salts. An intravenous infusion of 1 litre of 5 per cent dextrose followed by a litre of Hartmann's solution is set up to correct the ketosis and any electrolyte imbalance. She should then be maintained on an intravenous regimen of 3–4 litres per 24 hours. Serial electrolyte measurements are made on a daily basis until seen to be maintained at normal levels. Initially she is on nil by mouth until there has been no vomiting for 48 hours. Mouth washes will be required, and ice to suck is greatly appreciated.

Concurrent with the intravenous fluids, antiemetic therapy is also given.

> Although there are understandable concerns about giving any medication in early pregnancy, the well tried and tested antiemetic drugs are safer than uncontrolled vomiting.

Prochlorperazine (Stemetil) as a 5 mg suppository given 8-hourly is beneficial. (Be careful about giving higher doses of proclorperazine long term as Parkinsonian side-effects may occur.) If the vomiting persists, **promethazine** 25 mg may be given intramuscularly. Occasionally thyroid function tests may show a much higher T_4 level than is usual in pregnancy. Consultation with the physicians should be sought as treatment with carbimazole can be very helpful.

When the patient's condition has improved, oral fluids may be commenced, and if tolerated without further vomiting, the intravenous infusion can be discontinued. Gradually food is reintroduced until a relatively normal diet is possible. Thereafter, the dietary advice and antiemetic treatment is as for mild nausea and vomiting in pregnancy. The patient can then be discharged home, with clear instructions about the need for readmission should severe vomiting recur.

Urinary tract infections are the commonest cause, but vomiting can also be a feature of severe pregnancy-induced hypertension and acute hydramnios. A rarely seen, but often fatal, complication of pregnancy is acute fatty liver. It should be thought of as a possible diagnosis when malaise and vomiting is associated with abdominal pain in late pregnancy.

It is important not to forget the other common incidental causes of vomiting.

> Incidental causes of vomiting in pregnancy:
>
> (1) **gastroanteritis**; diarrhoea may also be a feature and it may have affected other members of the family;
>
> (2) **urinary tract infection/pyelonephritis**; an MSU will clarify the situation;
>
> (3) **acute appendicitis, intestinal obstruction**; these conditions can be notoriously difficult to diagnose in pregnancy and a surgical opinion must be obtained urgently if in any doubt;
>
> (4) **accident to an ovarian cyst or fibroid**; ultrasound may have already diagnosed the presence of these tumours before the onset of symptoms;
>
> (5) **intracranial tumours**; neurological examination will reveal signs of raised intracranial pressure.

118 Antenatal emergencies

When vomiting occurs late in pregnancy there is nearly always a pathological reason. This is also generally true of vomiting in the multiparous patient.

Termination of pregnancy is very rarely indicated and is only undertaken as a life-saving manoeuvre.

Major bleeding in early pregnancy

Until relatively recently, abortion was the major cause of maternal death due to haemorrhage, infection, and shock.

Very occasionally the degree of haemorrhage can be so severe that rather than simply agree with the GP's request to have the patient admitted even by ambulance, it is safer for the obstetric 'flying squad' to go to the patient, resuscitate and then bring her into hospital.

When haemorrhage is severe do not hesitate to call for help.

History, examination, and treatment of the woman go hand in hand. A history of the duration of the pregnancy and of recent events is obtained. She may have passed something other than blood, indicating a probable incomplete abortion. On examination, there may be signs of shock with a rapid pulse rate and low blood pressure. She may also be in considerable pain from uterine contractions and in great distress over the loss of the pregnancy. Abdominal examination is usually unremarkable. A sterile vaginal examination is important. The vagina can be ballooned out with clot and products of conception may be felt distending the cervical canal. Removal of this tissue either digitally or with sponge forceps can have a dramatic effect in improving her general condition and shock. Ergometrine 0.5 mg intramuscularly or 0.25 mg intravenously usually reduces the blood loss. Pethidine 100 mg or morphine 15 mg intramuscularly is given for the pain. Setting up an intravenous line in such circumstances can be difficult but is essential.

Blood is taken for a full blood count and for cross-matching. In cases of major haemorrhage, order at least 4 units of blood, warning the haematologist that more may be required. Evacuation of the uterus under general anaesthesia must now be considered unless ultrasonography shows that the uterine cavity is empty and the abortion process is complete.

Remember that retained clot has the same effect as retained products of conception.

If the patient is pyrexial and diagnosed as having a septic abortion, appropriate intravenous antibiotic therapy is commenced.

Haemorrhage breaks all the rules and must be stopped by means of curettage *even in the presence of obvious infection.*

These cases can be difficult for even the experienced operator. SEEK HELP.

Occasionally, major bleeding can occur during the second trimester. The presence of a low-lying placenta may already be known from the booking ultrasound examination. Remember that placenta praevia can reveal itself early and present as a major threat to abort. The management is initially conservative as described in the next section.

Antepartum haemorrhage

Owing to the increased chances of survival of extremely premature babies, the age of fetal viability has been lowered to 24 weeks. As a result, since October 1992, the time limits for stillbirth have been extended back to 24 weeks, which is also the limit for termination of pregnancy in the UK.

Following this change in definition of viability, antepartum haemorrhage (APH) is defined as bleeding from the genital tract after the 24th week of pregnancy and before the delivery of the baby. However, any vaginal bleeding after the 20th week generally has the same causes as APH and similar management.

The causes of APH include:

- placenta praevia
- abruptio placentae
- vaginal/cervical lesions:
    vaginal moniliasis
    vaginal varicosities
    cervical ectopy/ectropion
    cervical polypii
    cervical carcinoma
    trauma
- vasa praevia.

There is one absolute maxim in obstetrics:

> Every case of APH is regarded as being due to placenta praevia until proven otherwise.

Placenta praevia

Placenta praevia is defined as a placenta that is situated wholly or partially beneath the presenting part of the fetus. This therefore implies a variable degree of encroachment upon the lower segment of the uterus, the most major form covering the internal os of the cervix completely. Placenta praevia complicates less than 1 per cent of pregnancies.

In the UK the majority of potential cases of placenta praevia will have been found on ultrasound at booking or on detailed scanning at 18 weeks. When a woman is already known to have a low-lying placenta from her antenatal booking scan, she will have been warned to either avoid sexual intercourse altogether or at least avoid intercourse with deep penetration. The plan for such a patient would be to relocalize the placenta after the 28th week in the hope and expectation that with the further development and growth of the uterus, the placenta will have been drawn up out of its previous danger zone. She will have been given clear instructions to contact the labour ward immediately should *any* vaginal bleeding occur. It occasionally happens that a woman attending an antenatal clinic informs the staff of heavy vaginal bleeding that she had experienced the previous day. Unless immediate ultrasound facilities are available it can be difficult to 'persuade' the patient of the need to be admitted immediately. There may be problems of other children she has with her, the car on a meter, or her husband 'uncontactable'. All these obstacles can be overcome, but the importance of admission must be stressed and the risks of placenta praevia very clearly explained. While it must be borne in mind that the clinician's role is to inform and not to terrify the woman, turning taps on fully over the sink and indicating that haemorrhage can be of a similar degree, can be helpful in making the point to the reluctant patient!

While APH is the most dramatic way that placenta praevia can present, it can occasionally give non-haemorrhagic clues as to its presence.

> Placenta praevia must always be considered as a possible cause of unstable lie and a high head at term in the primigravida.

Characteristically, the APH due to placenta praevia is painless and is not usually associated with any physical activity apart from intercourse. Indeed, many APHs occur while the woman is asleep and she wakes up to find herself bleeding.

ALL cases of APH must be admitted to a hospital where there are facilities for Caesarean section.

Bleeding may be very slight and consist of only a few spots ('warning show') or may be a major haemorrhage of several units of blood. When the bleeding is only slight it is reasonable for the patient to be transported to hospital by ambulance but if the loss is heavy the obstetric 'flying squad' must be called out to assess the situation, set up an intravenous infusion, resuscitate if necessary and bring her into hospital. The alternative to the 'flying squad' is the Ambulance Paramedic Service where the staff have been trained in cardiopulmonary resuscitation and management of obstetric emergencies.

On examination the uterus is usually soft and non-tender. If the lie is longitudinal the presenting part is high, but the lie may be oblique with the presenting part in one of the iliac fossae. The fetal heart is present unless the degree of placental separation is major. (It is possible for a major (Grade IV) placenta praevia to be present when the head is engaged, if there is a succenturiate lobe of placenta attached to the lower segment beneath the head.)

UNDER NO CIRCUMSTANCES is a vaginal examination to be performed other than in an operating theatre with full facilities for immediate Caesarean section.

The patient who is actively bleeding is admitted to the labour ward for further assessment. Flying squad patients will already have an intravenous infusion set up and blood will have been taken for full blood count and cross-matching. If admission is from another source and she is still bleeding, she should be similarly treated.

It is perfectly reasonable for an experienced doctor to carry out a gentle speculum examination to determine whether or not the blood she is losing is coming through the cervical os and therefore presumably from the placental site.

If cervical pathology (polypii or ectopy) is seen, this is noted but does not influence the assumption that the patient has placenta praevia until proven otherwise.

Fetal well-being is determined by CTG.

If the pregnancy has reached 38 weeks, it is preferable to consider delivery of the baby. Examination under anaesthesia by an experienced obstetrician will confirm the diagnosis of placenta praevia and immediate Caesarean section can be performed.

The preterm patient is kept on the labour ward and observed until there has been no bleeding for 24 hours. If the placental site is not known, placental localization by ultrasound is then carried out. If placenta praevia is confirmed, the patient is managed by 'conservative expectant therapy'. This means that no intervention such as delivery is carried out at this stage. The patient is kept in hospital in the expectation of further APH. At least 'save serum' should be kept up-dated with the blood transfusion department, although for very major degrees of placenta praevia and APH it is best to have cross-matched blood readily available.

The morale of the woman often flags. She feels well and often requests a short escape for even 'just an hour or two', promising to 'do absolutely nothing' in the way of physical activity. These requests must be very sympathetically and firmly refused. She must be warned about the likelihood of a recurrent APH. If she were to haemorrhage at home, at best the settee or carpet will be ruined, at worst she or her baby may come to grief. If the demonstration with the taps has not already been carried out this would be a useful point to graphically portray what a major bleed can be like. (If, in spite of this, a patient insists upon taking her own discharge, the consultant must be informed and the patient asked to sign the appropriate self-discharge form). It is very important that both she and her partner fully understand the significance of placenta praevia and the plan of management.

Placental localization is carried out every 2–4 weeks in the hope that with the increasing growth of the uterus the placenta will be carried upwards. This is often the case with an anterior placenta as most of the uterine growth is over the anterior wall. A placenta praevia on the posterior uterine wall tends to remain praevia.

The intention is to get as close to 38 weeks as possible before delivery. The patient must be aware that she could have several 'excursions' to the labour ward before delivery is eventually decided upon. If a further APH does occur on the ward, an intravenous infusion is set up *before* she is transferred to the labour ward. Occasionally it is necessary to replace blood that is lost by transfusion. If at *any stage* of pregnancy bleeding is so heavy that replacement of blood is approaching 10 units or if the bleeding shows no sign of ceasing spontaneously, then delivery must be considered regardless of fetal chances of survival.

If by 38 weeks the placental site is known with accuracy and a major degree of placenta praevia has been diagnosed, there is no need to initially carry out an examination under anaesthesia. A lower segment Caesarean section should be performed by a skilled operator. *At least* 2 units of cross-matched blood should be available. The lower segment can be exceedingly vascular and the placenta itself may need to be incised or at least deflected in order to deliver the baby.

Because of this vascularity it is strongly advised that the operation should not be performed under epidural or spinal block but always under general anaesthetic. Surgical dexterity and speed is often required and the blood loss can be considerable and therefore very alarming to the conscious woman, as well as to her partner if he is in attendance at an epidural section.

For the woman who is being sterilized at delivery, and where the placenta praevia is anterior, there is sometimes a case for considering a classical Caesarean section so as to avoid the vascular lower segment.

The major complication at Caesarean section is **placenta accreta** (morbid adherence of the placenta). This seems to occur most commonly when there has been a previous Caesarean section scar to which the anterior placenta praevia is attached. Bleeding can be torrentially heavy and may even indicate the need for hysterectomy. **Postpartum haemorrhage** is relatively common owing to the generally poor musculature of the lower segment which has formed the placental bed. Occasionally such haemorrhage can be torrential. [For the management of major haemorrhage see PPH (p. 228).]

All cases of placenta praevia when there has been a previous Caesarean section MUST be performed by a consultant obstetrician.

If the diagnosis or degree of placerita praevia is uncertain, the aim should be to carry out an examination under anesthesia at 38 weeks, with the theatre staff standing by to proceed to immediate Caesarean section should bleeding be provoked or the placenta be felt through the vaginal fornices or cervix. If no bleeding is caused by the examination and the placenta cannot be felt, then forewater rupture by amniotomy is indicated. If heavy bleeding occurs subsequently, it is safest to proceed to Caesarean section. Occasionally the cervix is found to be unfavourable for amniotomy even though placenta praevia has been excluded. In such cases it is reasonable to proceed to 'ripen' the cervix with prostaglandins and reattempt amniotomy later. The patient should be pre-warned of this possibility.

In the Report on Confidential Enquiries into Maternal Deaths in the UK (1988–90), 5 of the 11 direct deaths caused by antepartum haemorrhage were due to placenta praevia. Care was considered to be substandard in all 5 cases. In four cases who underwent Caesarean section, the operation was performed by the unsupervised registrar. The report stresses the need for both elective and emergency Caesarean section for placenta praevia to be carried out by, or directly supervised by, a consultant obstetrician.

Abruptio placentae

APH from abruptio placentae is due to the separation of a normally situated placenta. Abruptio placentae complicates up to 2 per cent of pregnancies.

Although many cases of placental abruption have no apparent cause, the incidence is higher among multiparous patients and in pregnancies complicated by either essential hypertension or PIH. When amniotomy is carried out in cases of polyhydramnios, the sudden decompression of the over-distended uterus can lead to a 'shearing off' of the placenta from its site of attachment. Very occasionally there is a traumatic cause such as external cephalic version or a blow to the abdomen.

In placenta praevia, the placenta is very close to, if not over, the internal os of the cervix. As a result the inevitable APH associated with a low-lying placenta is immediately revealed. In contrast, the APH following the abruption of a normally situated upper segment placenta may at first be concealed and very strong contractions can result.

> ALWAYS think of abruptio placentas as the cause of *spontaneous* hypertonic contractions.

Blood loss will only be revealed when blood from the abruption site eventually escapes between the membranes and uterine wall.

Minor abruptio placentae

The presenting feature in abruption is usually the sudden onset of abdominal pain, owing to blood released at the site of placental separation being forced between uterine muscle fibres. In minor cases of abruption the pain may be quite slight with only minimal uterine tenderness, and no revealed bleeding ever occurs. Ultrasonography may be able to show the presence of a haematoma between the placenta and uterine wall. (Sometimes the evidence of abruption is only confirmed after delivery when the placenta is found to be indented by an old blood clot.)

> Abruptio placentae must always been included in the differential diagnosis of ? cause of abdominal pain and uterine tenderness.

Minor degrees of abruption may occur from the placental edge and present as a painless APH. The woman will be admitted and managed initially as a case of placenta praevia, but subsequent ultrasonography will reveal a normally sited placenta. Unless there are other concerns for maternal and fetal well-being such as PIH or progression of the pregnancy beyond 37 weeks, such patients are usually allowed to go home after there has been no further blood loss for 48 hours. However, these pregnancies must be regarded as being 'high risk', owing to a probable reduction in placental efficiency due to placental scarring at the site of the marginal abruption. Close fetal monitoring by serial ultrasound, kick chart, and CTG are essential. Delivery should be considered at 38 weeks as the perinatal mortality rate (PNM) is increased if left to go to term or beyond.

Moderate/severe abruptio placentae

The patient will present with a history of sudden severe onset of abdominal pain. As there is a major degree of placental separation, the blood loss is greater and is therefore likely to be revealed. Hypovolaemic shock is a frequent feature and its severity may be totally out of proportion to the apparently small amount of blood that has been revealed. On even gentle palpation the uterus is tender and often board-like. It can be very difficult to palpate fetal parts. If the baby is still alive, there are usually signs of fetal distress.

The initial emergency management is to resuscitate the patient *before* transferring her to hospital by 'flying squad' or Ambulance Paramedic Service. Intravenous morphine 10 mg will relieve severe pain. During the setting up of an intravenous infusion, blood is taken for cross-matching, Kleihauer testing if rhesus-negative, and for coagulation studies. Hartmann's solution can be commenced prior to giving blood. The 'flying squad' will carry Group O rhesus-negative blood which will need to be given rapidly.

On arrival at the labour ward, at least 4 units of blood must be cross-matched and an urgent coagulation profile requested. An indwelling bladder catheter is required to monitor urine output. There is always the risk of oliguria in the under-perfused patient.

A central venous pressure line is essential in order to avoid the easily committed error of *under-transfusing* the patient.

Hypofibrinogenaemia with an associated loss of platelets is a common feature of severe cases of abruption. Severe **disseminated intravascular coagulation** (DIC) may indicate an urgent need for fresh blood, fresh platelets, fresh frozen plasma, and other blood products. It is important that the haematologist and blood transfusion department are kept fully informed of the clinical situation.

The fetal mortality in cases of abruptio placentas can be as high as 100 per cent.

In view of this, if the baby is still alive, the need for delivery is urgent and is best achieved by immediate Caesarean section. This should be the method of choice even in the absence of fetal distress unless vaginal delivery seems imminent. The Caesarean section should only be performed by an experienced obstetrician, as it can be extremely difficult. The extravasation of blood into the myometrium produces the appearance of the typical Couvelaire uterus which appears to be covered with small petechial haemorrhages beneath the serosa. Haemostasis can be extraordinarily difficult to achieve.

Occasionally the clinical situation will produce a dilemma for the obstetrician. The presence of a coagulopathy adds to the maternal problem and can discourage operative intervention. Once fetal distress is severe, the fetal outlook is poor even if the fetus is delivered alive by Caesarean section. Yet even in this situation, a Caesarean section still offers the only prospect of delivering a live baby.

If the baby is already dead, it is fortunately rare to have to resort to Caesarean section. The only indication would be uncontrollable haemorrhage. If contractions are already well established, amniotomy in the operating theatre is advisable. A syntocinon infusion should always be set up. Labour is usually rapid. As the oedematous, bruised uterus is less efficient at contracting during the third stage, intravenous ergometrine 0.25 mg is given and the syntocinon infusion is continued.

DO NOT RELAX VIGILANCE AFTER DELIVERY.

Postpartum haemorrhage is the major problem and can be fatal. There is a temptation to over-transfuse and here again the central venous pressure line is invaluable. Urine output is closely watched. Oliguria and even renal failure can further complicate the situation. [For the management of major haemorrhage see PPH (p. 228).]

In severe cases of abruption, the intensive combined efforts of obstetrician, anaesthetist, haematologist, and renal physician are required to reduce the risk of a maternal death.

In the Report on Confidential Enquiries into Maternal Deaths by in UK (1988–90), 5 of the 11 direct deaths caused by antepartum haemorrhage were due to abruptio placentae. Care was considered to be substandard in 4 cases, but in two of these the patient had no access to medical assistance. In one case, severe anaemia and a coagulation defect complicated the abruption and in the second case the Ceasarean section had been delegated to a senior house officer.

Do not forget the risk of rhesus iso-immunization in the rhesus-negative woman. The transplacental haemorrhage can be large and an adequate dosage of anti-D immunoglobulin is important.

Incidental causes of antepartum haemorrhage

Placenta praevia will need to be excluded as a potential cause of antepartum haemorrhage before a vaginal or cervical cause (p. 119) can be definitely accepted as the source of blood loss. With the exception of cervical carcinoma, bleeding is rarely heavy (p. 70). The diagnosis of vaginal or cervical pathology is made by speculum examination.

Vasa praevia is a rare problem which occurs when the vessels of the umbilical cord lie over the internal os of the cervix, having separated from each other some distance away from their velamentous insertion into the placenta or into a succenturiate lobe. The vessels run freely in the membranes and as such are more vulnerable to injury. Spontaneous rupture of cord vessels late in pregnancy or in labour, or rupture at amniotomy, can produce a brisk 'show' and rapidly leads to exsanguination of the fetus.

It is essential that haemorrhage from a fetal source is recognized rapidly. Changes in the fetal heart rate associated with even a small, fresh, vaginal blood loss must suggest a diagnosis of vasa praevia.

> When bleeding occurs at amniotomy, the blood must be tested for fetal haemoglobin urgently.

If the vaginal bleeding is confirmed as being fetal in origin, an emergency Caesarean section is carried out.

Imminent eclampsia and eclampsia

Imminent elampsia

Severe proteinuric pregnancy-induced hypertension is asymptomatic unless eclampsia is imminent.

> Symptoms suggesting imminent eclampsia:
>
> - headaches
> - blurring of vision
> - epigastric pain
> - vomiting.

Associated with the onset of significant symptoms is the development of further clinical signs.

Signs suggesting imminent eclampsia:

- rapid rise in diastolic blood pressure, > 105
- hyper-relexia with ankle clonus
- increasing proteinuria
- decreased urine output.

If there is a suspicion that eclampsia is imminent it is essential that this is treated as an emergency. If the patient is at home, the Ambulance Paramedic Service may elect to call out the 'flying squad' so that adequate anticonvulsant and hypotensive therapy can be achieved *before* transfer to hospital with an experienced obstetrician in attendance. It is equally important to achieve the same degree of control before transfer from an antenatal ward to the labour ward. An eclamptic fit while in the lift *en route* to the labour ward is then less likely to occur.

It must be remembered that hypotensive therapy alone will not prevent eclampsia.

Treatment must always be a combination of hypotensive and anticonvulsant:

Diazepam (diazemuls) 10 mg intravenously as a bolus followed by 40 mg in 500 ml of Hartmann's solution transfused slowly until the patient is drowsy. Once on the labour ward the diazepam can be administered via a syringe pump (40 mg in 40 ml).

Hydralazine 5–10 mg intravenously as a bolus followed by 40 mg in 500 ml of Hartmann's solution titrated against the blood pressure to maintain the diastolic below 100 mmHg. Once on the labour ward the hydralazine can be administered via a syringe pump, 1 mg per ml starting at 1 ml per hour.

Once in hospital, an alternative drug therapy involves the use of phenytoin (which may be more effective than diazepam at preventing eclamptic fits) and labetalol to control the hypertension. There is also a growing interest in the use of nifedipine, although its use is as yet unlicensed in pregnancy.

Phenytoin is given intravenously via a syringe pump a dosage of 15 mg per kg over a period of 30 minutes: i.e., the dosage is 750 mg if he maternal weight is <70 kg, 1000 mg if 70–90 kg and 1250 mg if >90 km. (The phenytoin is diluted with saline NOT dextrose so as to avoid crystalization. Continuous ECG monitoring is recommended as marked bradycardia and hypotension may occur if administered faster than 50 mg per minute. After 8 hours a further dose of 500 mg is given by pump. Then 100 mg intravenously or orally 8-hourly for 72 hours.

Labetalol is given intravenously as a 20 mg bolus over a period of 2 minutes. Then 200 mg in 50 ml saline is administered via a syringe pump. The rate of infusion is then titrated against the blood pressure, aiming to maintain a diastolic pressure between 90 and 100.

Nifedipine 20 mg given as a *slow* intravenous bolus brings about a smooth, rapid reduction in blood pressure. After a 6-hour interval, 10–20 mg orally 12-hourly is effective. CAUTION. There can be profound hypotension when added to a beta-blocker or methyl dopa.

The blood pressure is recorded at 15-minute intervals. Fluid input and output is monitored. The intravenous infusions are administered via a 16 gauge cannula. No more than one litre 12-hourly is given. Urine output is measured hourly via an indwelling Foley catheter and urimeter. If the urine output falls below 30 ml per hour, a central venous pressure line should be set up by the anaesthetist, preferably using an ante-cubital vein. An intravenous, infusion of 500 ml of human albumin solution 4.5 per cent or 200 ml of 20 per cent mannitol may be required to promote a diuresis.

Fetal well-being is observed by continuous CTG.

Blood is taken for a full blood count, platelets, coagulation profile, urea, and electrolytes. This is repeated 12-hourly.

Once the condition has stabilized, delivery of the baby is the only cure. Conservative management after 34 weeks is pointless. Occasionally, imminent eclampsia can occur as early as 26 weeks and, unfortunately, the baby will have to take its chances. Vaginal delivery would only be considered if the cervix was favourable, preferably in a multiparous patient. The presentation should be cephalic and there should be no evidence of intrauterine growth retardation or abnormal CTG.

An epidural should be used for analgesia and to assist in control of the blood pressure as long as the platelet level is greater than 150×10^9. **Disseminated intravascular coagulation (DIC)** is a contraindication to using an epidural. If the platelet level is below 150, excellent analgesia can be achieved with diamorphine 10 mg by intramuscular injection.

In view of the increased possibility of Caesarean section, ranitidine 150 mg orally 6-hourly is indicated.

Once in the second stage of labour, delivery must not involve maternal effort. An elective forceps or ventouse delivery is indicated. Syntocinon 5–10 units intravenously should always be used in the third stage of labour instead of products containing ergometrine.

> DO NOT RELAX VIGILANCE POSTNATALLY. 30 per cent of eclamptic fits occur in the first 48 hours of the puerperium.

Caesarean section is the safer option in a deteriorating situation, in the primigravida, unfavourable cervix, abnormal presentations, IUGR, and gross prematurity. (See HELLP syndrome p. 230).

Eclampsia

For 20 per cent of the women who develop eclampsia there is no warning sign or symptom, all previous blood pressure recordings being normal and no proteinuria being detected. For the majority, there are prodromal signs and symptoms of imminent eclampsia. Fifty per cent of eclamptic fits occur antenatally, 20 per cent during labour and the remainder in the puerperium, usually within 48 hours of delivery.

> The essential emergency management of an eclamptic fit is to maintain an airway and to stop the convulsion.

The immediate management of eclampsia includes:

(1) CALL FOR HELP!
(2) the patient must be turned on to her side into the recovery position, while restraining her to prevent self-injury;
(3) the angle of the jaw is elevated and an airway established and maintained;
(4) suction may be required;
(5) oxygen is given by face mask (intubation/ventilation may be needed);
(6) to stop the convulsion, **diazepam** (Diazemuls 10–30 mg is given intravenously as a bolus;
(7) to control the hypertension, **hydralazine** or **labetalol** as for imminent eclampsia is administered;
(8) in labour, an epidural will have the advantage of both relieving pain which may trigger further convulsions, and reducing the diastolic blood pressure.

> If eclampsia occurs antenatally or in labour, delivery of the baby is the only safe action. To delay delivery to try and 'buy time' is simply to risk further convulsions.

If the cervix is unfavourable or if there are signs of fetal distress, an emergency Caesarean section must be carried out once the situation is under control. Thereafter the management is as described for imminent eclampsia.

Hypertension is now the chief direct cause of maternal death in UK. In the Report on Confidential Enquiries into Maternal Deaths in the UK (1988–90), there were 27 cases where pregnancy-induced hypertension and eclampsia were the sole causes of death. In 25 cases the blood pressure was normal in early pregnancy. There were 14 deaths from eclampsia.

It is also significant the hypertensive disorders of pregnancy featured in 17 other deaths, although the hypertension itself was not the direct cause of death. Furthermore, it was noted that 18 (41 per cent) of the patients whose direct or indirect deaths were associated with adult respiratory distress syndrome (ARDS), had hypertensive disorder of pregnancy.

Substandard care featured in 24 (89 per cent) of the 27 deaths. There was delay or failure in obtaining GP referral in five cases. In 17 cases the substandard care was the responsibility of the consultant obstetric unit alone. There was delay in making clinical decisions in that appropriate hypotensive therapy was given too late or delivery deferred too long. There was a lack of awareness by junior medical and midwifery staff of the importance of the appropriate antepartum, intrapartum, and postpartum management of the hypertensive patient with or without proteinuria. Involvement of the consultant staff was often left too late. The message is loud and clear. **Do not treat hypertensive disorders of pregnancy casually. The consequences could be lethal.**

Preterm (premature) labour

It is generally accepted that labour is preterm if it occurs before the 37th week. This will complicate up to 10 per cent of births, 2 per cent occuring before 32 weeks. It is still a major cause of perinatal death.

> For up to 45 per cent of preterm labours no obvious cause can be found.

Preterm labour may be a spontaneous event or may be the result of premature induction of labour when it is considered that the risks to either the mother or the fetus are too great to safely allow the pregnancy to continue any further. It will be seen below that a number of the causes of preterm labour are interrelated. For example, low socio-economic class and smoking may lead to IUGR and premature induction.

Causes of preterm labour

Maternal causes
- young maternal age
- low-socioeconomic class
- smoking
- previous preterm labour
- pyrexia (pyelonephritis)
- ill health
- following surgery (appendicectomy)
- premature induction of labour for a variety of causes, especially severe PIH, IUGR

Uterine causes
- cervical incompetence
- uterine abnormalities (congenital and acquired)

Feto-placental causes
- a multiple pregnancy
- polyhydramnios
- anterpartum haemorrhage:
    placenta praevia
    abruptio placentas
- intrauterine death
- fetal abnormality
- placental insufficiency
- premature spontaneous rupture of membranes.

Is she really in labour?

The diagnosis of preterm labour is often difficult. Many women are admitted in labour, and it is only subsequently that it becomes apparent that painful Braxton Hicks contractions are being experienced.

Admission to hospital is the only safe option.

Vaginal examination to assess cervical dilatation and external cardiotocography should reveal the true state of affairs. If there is doubt, as is often the case, the patient should be kept in hospital for further assessment. If contractions become more frequent, the vaginal examination is, repeated. If symptoms subside, she should at least stay in hospital overnight and have a further vaginal assessment the next day. If the findings are unchanged and there is no other obstetric reason for the woman to remain an in-patient, she can be discharged home. It is always worth while to arrange for a high vaginal swab and a mid-stream urine (MSU) collection to be sent for culture. An immediate report can be given on the the white cell count in the MSU and the likelihood of infection.

Monoclonal antibody tests are becoming established which may dramatically improve the diagnosis of imminent preterm labour. The basis of these tests is the detection of the protein fibronectin in cervical mucus. It has been shown that the presence of fibronectin during the 24th–34th weeks is a useful marker for the onset of preterm labour. If detected, appropriate intervention therapy can be considered. Conversely, if fibronectin is *not* detected, the woman may be allowed to return home.

Established preterm labour

Labour is considered to be established if painful contractions are occuring regularly at least every 10 minutes and the cervix is effaced and found to be 2 cm or more dilated with bulging membranes during contractions.

> ALWAYS discuss the management of these cases with the Senior Registrar or Consultant.

If preterm labour occurs before 34 weeks, most centres will attempt to suppress labour, as long as there are no contraindications. This should apply regardless of the degree of dilatation of the cervix **as long as the membranes are intact**:

> *Contraindications to the suppression of labour:*
>
> - ruptured membranes
> - chorioamnionitis
> - IUGR
> - fetal abnormality
> - fetal distress
> - antepartum haemorrhage
> - maternal conditions:
>   diabetes
>   hypertension
>   cardiac or thyroid disease.

If it is decided to attempt to suppress labour, the preparation most commonly used is the beta-sympathomimetic drug ritodrine. Ritodrine needs to be given by slow intravenous infusion to have any chance of being effective.

Ritodrine: A controlled infusion syringe pump should be used if possible. The concentration of ritodrine should be 3 mg per ml [150 mg of ritodrine solution (15 ml) is added to 35 ml of 5 per cent dextrose to make up a volume of 50 ml.]

The pump is set at 1 ml per hour (50 μg per minute) and the rate is increased by 0.5 ml per hour every 10 minutes until:

- contractions stop, or
- maternal pulse rate reaches 140 per minute, or
- fetal tachycardia >180 per minute, or
- there is a significant change in maternal systolic blood pressure

It is therefore essential to monitor the fetal heart rate and contractions with continuous CTG. The maternal pulse and blood pressure are assessed at 15-minute intervals while increasing the drip rate, and thereafter every 30 minutes. The patient's lung bases are checked 12-hourly. Blood urea, electrolytes, and glucose levels are checked 12-hourly.

Rare fatal cases of maternal pulmonary oedema have been reported in association with the use of ritodrine.

The use of a syringe pump will keep the volume of fluid at a minimum, as fluid overload is the most important single factor in causing pulmonary oedema. Saline should be avoided except in diabetics.

The aim is to continue with the ritodrine for 12 hours after contractions cease, possibly reducing the rate of infusion. There should be an overlap of oral ritodrine 10 mg 30 minutes before the intravenous route is stopped. Ritodrine can then be continued orally at 10 mg 2-hourly for 24 hours before reducing to 10 mg 4- to 8-hourly long term.

If the cervix is not more than 2 cm dilated, 80 per cent of premature labours can be suppressed.

Even when the cervix is as much as 6 cm dilated, it is possible to consider a 'rescue' cervical cerclage **but only if contractions can be completely suppressed**. There is, after all, nothing to lose, since if the 'rescue' attempt fails the patient will be no worse off and at least will know that everything possible has been done to try to prolong the pregnancy in order to gain maturity. It is, however, a difficult procedure to carry out with a high failure rate. The patient must be advised about the risks of membrane rupture occurring during the procedure and of subsequent delivery.

A 'rescue' cerclage under these circumstances should only be carried out by an experienced obstetrician.

Under general anaesthesia, the patient is placed in lithotomy in a steep head-down Trendellenberg position. She is cleaned, draped, and catheterized. A single-bladed speculum is inserted into the vagina and the degree of cervical dilatation determined. Sponge-holding forceps are placed around the edge of the dilated cervix. The 30 ml balloon of a self-retaining catheter is filled with sterile water and the catheter tip excised. The balloon is used to gently replace the membranes back into the uterine cavity. Gentle shaking of the sponge holders can assist (Fig. 4.1.). Once the membranes are replaced, the cervix is closed, preferably with four nylon sutures (Fig. 4.2.), which have the effect of flattening the cervix and increasing the degree of support to the pregnancy.

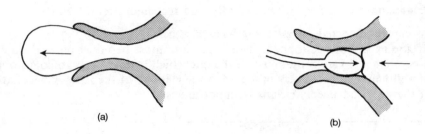

(a)   (b)

Fig. 4.1   (a) Diagram to show membranes bulging through dilated cervix; (b) After 'shaking' the membranes back into the uterus using several sponge holding forceps around the cervix, the membranes are held in position by the balloon of a Foley catheter (with the tip excised). Sutures can now be sited.

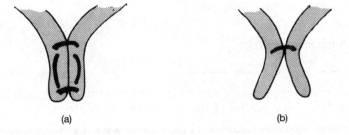

(a)   (b)

Fig. 4.2   (a) Diagram to show the placing of 4 No. 1 nylon sutures which have the effect of flattening the entire cervix and thereby increasing the support given to the area of the internal os; (b) Diagram to show the site of the standard single cervical cerclage which gives solitary support to the internal os.

There is little point in trying to suppress labour after 34 weeks' gestation, or if the membranes have ruptured.

There will, however, be exceptions to these general guidelines, such as a very poor past obstetric history, the need to try to 'buy time' for dexamethasone therapy to become effective to aid lung maturity or to attempt to stop labour prior to *in utero* transfer to a centre with better facilities for dealing with very small preterm babies.

Many units will use steroids to increase the production of lung surfactant and thereby reduce the incidence of respiratory distress syndrome. Steroids are contraindicated after 34 weeks and in the presence of severe hypertension.

Steroid regimens include:

Dexamethasone 12 mg intramuscularly and repeated after 12 hours.

Betamethasone 12 mg intramuscularly and repeated after 24 hours.

(This can be repeated on a weekly basis if necessary.)

If labour cannot be stopped, then a decision must be taken on the route of delivery. The delivery route must be the one which is least likely to compromise fetal well-being and is largely based upon the viability of the fetus. Consultation with the neonatal paediatricians is important.

> Caesarean section should not be carried out for fetal interests before the 26th week.

The chief indications for an elective Caesarean section are:

- any presentation other than cephalic
- fetal distress
- antepartum haemorrhage.

> Always remember that an elective Caesarean section is no guarantee of a live baby and may not be in the best maternal interests.

If vaginal delivery of a viable baby is planned, the presentation must be cephalic, without signs of fetal distress or antepartum haemorrhage. An epidural should be considered and fetal well-being monitored with continuous CTG. At delivery an elective episiotomy is indicated. Fetal distress is an indication for delivery of the baby by the speediest route, i.e. forceps if the cervix is fully dilated and Caesarean section if not yet in the second stage of labour.

Premature rupture of membranes (PROM) without contractions

Premature rupture of membranes is associated with cord prolapse and the risk of ascending infection. The diagnosis is confirmed by a sterile speculum examination. It is usually easy to recognize the pool of liquor between the blades of the speculum or in the posterior fornix of the vagina. When the amount of liquor seen is minimal, the diagnosis is confirmed by noting the colour change of a sterile nitrazine swab from orange to purple. A high vaginal swab is taken for culture.

Unless there is an indication to deliver the baby, PROM without contractions is best managed conservatively. The chief indication for delivery is evidence of infection.

> AVOID DIGITAL VAGINAL EXAMINATION unless induction of labour is intended.

Occasionally a woman with very early PROM will continue to trickle and/or intermittently gush liquor vaginally for several weeks. This situation does not contraindicate the use of steroids. Indeed there may be a need to consider the use of ritodrine, in spite of there being ruptured membranes, in order to 'buy time' both for steroids to be of benefit to try to gain further maturity by discouraging the onset of contractions. No action needs to be taken until evidence of infection is found. This should then be treated vigorously. It is debatable whether or not the prophylactic use of antibiotics is of any benefit. A risk to the fetus of prolonged PROM is lung hypoplasia.

5   Induction of labour

Improvements in monitoring fetal well-being have reduced the incidence of intervention in modern obstetric practice. However, induction of labour must be considered if it is felt that delivery is in the best interests of either the mother or the baby, or both.

> The guiding principal must be SAFETY.

If it is safer for the baby to be delivered than to remain *in utero*, then delivery is the only option. If continuation of the pregnancy should significantly threaten the health of the mother then delivery is indicated regardless of the maturity of the baby.

The major indications for induction of labour

- postmaturity
- fetal conditions:
  IUGR
  antenatal fetal distress
  twins
  rhesus iso-immunization
  intrauterine death
  lethal fetal abnormality
- maternal conditions:
  PIH and essential hypertension
  diabetes
  APH
  poor obstetric history.

The decision to induce labour must be based on sound obstetric practice and not be the result of patient pressure or social convenience. ALWAYS explain to the woman the reason for induction; many will be apprehensive at this apparent interference in their pregnancy.

A Caesarean section resulting from a failed induction must never cause the obstetrician to regret the earlier decision to intervene.

If labour itself should further compromise fetal well-being, then delivery must be by elective Caesarean section. However, Caesarean section would be contraindicated if there was gross prematurity (before 26 weeks), as the mother would be subjected to major surgery with little chance of fetal survival.

Contraindications to the induction of labour

- social requirements/convenience
- cephalo-pelvic disproportion
- previous failed trial of labour
- two or more previous Caesarean sections
- previous classical Caesarean section
- major degree of placenta praevia
- major abruptio placentae with a live baby
- cord presentation
- certain malpresentations
    transverse lie
    brow
    breech plus complications
- elderly primigravida plus complications
- fetus severely compromised by IUGR or severe antenatal fetal distress.

If labour is to be induced, it is important that the induction attempt should succeed. It can be demoralizing to both the woman and her partner if the induction should fail. The likelihood of this happening can be determined by the Bishop score which gives an 'inducibility rating' (see Table 5.1).

A Bishop score of 5 or more is likely to result in a successful induction attempt.

The 'unfavourable' cervix

It frequently happens that there are indications to induce labour when the Bishop score is very low. Under these circumstances it is highly likely that an attempt at normal induction methods will fail. 'Ripening' of the cervix can be obtained with the use of vaginal prostaglandin E_2 (PGE_2) either as a tablet or gel.

Table 5.1   Bishop score for status of the cervix

SCORE	0	1	2	3
Dilation (cm)	0	1–2	3–4	5+
Length of cervix (cm)	3	2	1	0
Station	−3	−2	−1	+1, +2
Consistency	firm	medium	soft	
Position	posterior	mid	anterior	

Score each component, then add scores for total Bishop score

If the cervix is assessed the night before the planned induction and found to be unfavourable, a 3 mg tablet or 1–2 mg of gel is placed into the posterior fornix of the vagina. Care should be taken not to apply any lubricating cream onto the tablet as this can interfere with absorption. An external CTG transducer is used to monitor the fetal heart rate during the next half-hour. It is frequently necessary to repeat the PGE_2 the next morning if the cervix is still unfavourable. However, a significant proportion of these patients will labour spontaneously and progress naturally as a result of the first PGE_2 insertion.

If cervical ripening is being performed on a compromised baby (IUGR), it may be safer to delay the PGE_2 insertion until the morning, when there will be a fuller obstetric team available on the labour ward unit. Continuous fetal heart monitoring is essential in this situation.

Extra-amniotic FGE_2 can be administered via a Foley catheter inserted into the uterine cavity and anchored above the internal os by the inflated balloon of the catheter. This is a highly successful method of induction should PGE_2 tablets fail. After 6 hours of extra-amniotic infusion the PGE_2 is stopped and 1 hour later syntocinon is given by intravenous infusion. This must be used carefully in view of the synergistic action between prostaglandins and oxytocin. The catheter falls out of the cervix at 3 cm dilatation when a fore-water membrane rupture can easily be performed. (See Fig. 5.1.)

Surgical induction of labour

When the Bishop score is satisfactory, the lie is longitudinal, and the presenting part is not high, amniotomy or artificial rupture of the membranes (ARM) is generally accepted as the method of choice for induction of labour. This should only be performed in a labour ward environment where there are emergency facilities available for coping with any complication that may arise. ARM is a potent method of inducing labour and has the advantage of revealing the presence of meconium in the liquor and also permits access to the fetus for both efficient fetal heart rate monitoring via a scalp clip and fetal blood sampling.

If the cervix is found to be unfavourable, the temptation to continue with the ARM and force an amnihook through a tight unfavourable cervix must be resisted. PGE_2 'ripening' should be undertaken first.

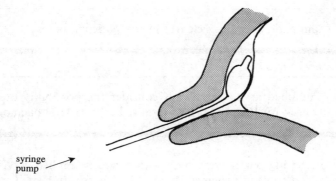

syringe
pump

Fig. 5.1 Extra-amniotic prostaglandin induction of labour. The balloon of the Foley catheter is shown above the level of the internal os of the cervix, lying between the membranes and uterine wall.

Fore-water rupture

Using an aseptic technique, a vaginal examination is carried out. One of the two examining fingers is gently inserted through the dilated cervical os and a gentle membrane sweep is performed. An amnihook is guided between the fingers. The finger within the cervix is then used to press the back of the amnihook against the membranes over the fetal scalp so as to allow the hook to snare the membranes. The amnihook is gently withdrawn while maintaining gentle pressure against the membranes over the scalp. Release of liquor generally follows. The volume and colour of the liquor is noted. The gap in the membranes can then be enlarged by the examining finger. A scalp clip can be applied for fetal ECG. The fetal heart rate must be checked after ARM. (See Table 5.2.)

Table 5.2 Example of a Vaginal Examination stamp which could be entered into the notes at each V.E.

Vaginal examination Date .... **Time** ....
Indication ....
Cervix .... Dilation .... Length ....
Membranes ....

Fetus
Presentation .... Position ....
Flexion .... Station ....
Caput .... Moulding ....
Pelvis ....
Conclusion ....

Signature ....

> Enter all examination findings clearly in the patient's notes.

> If blood is obtained at ARM, always consider the possibility of a vasa praevia and check for the presence of fetal red cells or fetal haemoglobin.

When the presenting part is very high with a poorly applied cervix, ARM is more likely to lead to cord prolapse. If an ARM is still indicated, this should be carried out in the labour ward theatre where there are immediate facilities for emergency Caesarean section.

Hind-water rupture

This method of amniotomy used to be advocated in the presence of polyhydramnios or when the presenting part was high.

A metal Drew-Smythe catheter was passed through the cervix and curved behind the fetal head. On introducing the metal plunger within the catheter the membranes over the hind-waters in the area of the fetal neck were ruptured and released through the hollow catheter. In theory, and sometimes in practice, this would permit a more controlled release of liquor. However, sometimes the membranes would not rupture at all and often the fore-waters ruptured as well. In addition, unless the placental site was known with accuracy, there was the risk of disturbing the placenta and obtaining a 'bloody tap' instead of liquor. Generally the use of hind-water rupture has fallen into disrepute.

Medical induction of labour

PGE$_2$ tablets or gel can be used not only to 'ripen' the otherwise unfavourable cervix and so initiate labour, but will also very effectively induce labour when the cervix is favourable. This is then followed by amniotomy. The use of drugs alone to induce labour is rarely employed in modern obstetrics.

Sometimes it is decided to induce labour maximally by means of ARM and immediate syntocinon infusion. The alternative is to assess the effect of ARM and several hours later augment labour with additional intravenous syntocinon if progress is considered to be unsatisfactory.

Intravenous syntocinon infusion.
1.   Two units of syntocinon are added to 500 ml of 5% dextrose or Hartmann's solution. The infusion is commenced at 10 drops per minute (2.6 mU per minute) and doubled every 15 minutes until regular contractions are established. The drip set can be regulated by an infusion pump which incorporates a drop counter. If contractions remain inadequate the strength of syntocinon in the infusion can be increased.

2.   An alternative method of administering syntocinon is to use a syringe pump. 15 units of syntocinon are added to 50 ml of 5% dextrose or Hartmann's solution. The syringe is set at 0.5 ml per hour (2.5 mU per minute) and increased by 0.5 ml every 15 minutes up to a maximum of 5.5 ml per hour (27.5 mU per minute).

When contractions are satisfactory, occurring at a rate of approximately one in every 3 minutes and lasting for 45 seconds, the infusion rate can be reduced as long as contractions are maintained.

Complications of induction

Failed induction

This is more likely to occur in preterm inductions or when the Bishop score is low and no ripening has been undertaken with PGE_2. If uterine action cannot be improved so that delivery will occur within 24 hours of amniotomy, Caesarean section will be the only solution.

Cord prolapse

This should be a rare complication of induction. If before induction the cord is presenting, ARM is absolutely contraindicated until the cord is no longer in this danger zone. If the need to deliver is urgent in this situation, an elective Caesarean section will be safer.

In the presence of, polyhydramnios the cord can be washed down in a gush of liquor at ARM.

If the presenting part is high, the cord can prolapse even though there was no obvious cord presentation before ARM.

When the presenting part is a poor fit in the pelvis as with a flexed breech or footling breech, the cord can snake down between the fetal legs. Indeed a footling presentation is an indication for an elective Caesarean section.

Abruptio placentae

This complication can occur due to shearing off of the placenta from its site if there is a sudden decompression of the uterus at amniotomy in the presence of extreme polyhydramnios.

Abruption may also complicate attempts at hind-water rupture.

Acute fetal distress

The sudden decompression of the uterus at amniotomy when there is polyhydramnios, can lead to a 'crimping' of the placental site and reduction in placental blood flow. The effects on the fetal heart rate can be dramatic.

Ascending infection

This is unlikely to complicate labour unless the interval between ARM and delivery is greater than 24 hours. Infection can occasionally become established in considerably less time than this. (It is for this very reason that a digital vaginal examination is avoided when there has been premature rupture of membranes.) If there are pathogens in the vagina, especially group B beta-haemolytic streptococci before ARM, ascending infection leading to amnionitis and fetal pneumonia can prove to be fatal for the baby. Signs of maternal pyrexia or of offensive liquor demand vigorous antibiotic therapy.

Prematurity

This will be an unavoidable consequence of premature induction of labour whether indicated for fetal or maternal well-being.

If the dates have been incorrectly calculated, induction for apparent postmaturity may lead to prematurity simply because the dates are wrong.

Hypertonic contractions

Syntocinon can cause hypertonic uterine activity when the contractions can run into each other with little respite in between. It is important not to blindly increase the rate of a syntocinon infusion quarter-hourly when contractions are already satisfactory. The syntocinon rate should be titrated to the degree of uterine activity which usually means that the infusion rate can be reduced once labour is definitely established. Occasionally a tetanic contraction may occur lasting for several minutes causing marked fetal hypoxia.

Syntocinon, if used at all in the 'grand multip', must be used with extreme caution owing to the dramatically increased sensitivity of the uterus to oxytocin.

It must also be remembered that PGE_2 will enhance the action of syntocinon given subsequently.

Uterine rupture

This is an extremely rare complication in the primigravida. Among multipara, tonic contractions due to syntocinon can lead to uterine rupture especially if there has been previous scarring from Caesarean section.

PGE_2 is effective in cervical ripening, probably by changing the consistency of cervical collagen. If cervical ripening is indicated for a patient who has had a previous Caesarean section, it may be considered safer to deliver her once more by Caesarean section rather than risk a similar process occurring in the uterine scar.

Water intoxication

This is unlikely to occur in any labour of normal duration where normal quantities of syntocinon have been used. It has very occasionally been seen in very prolonged labours where there have been high-volume infusions of electrolyte-free fluid in the presence of high concentrations of syntocinon. In cases of prolonged labour, syntocinon administered by syringe pump will considerably reduce this risk.

Induction in special cases

Breech induction

There should not be any problem in the induction of labour for a frank breech with extended legs as the shape of the presenting part forms a snug fit in the pelvis. Amniotomy should not present any problem as long as the breech is engaged in the pelvis.

When the breech is in a flexed position, the shape of the presenting part is not ideal and it is possible for the cord to be entangled with the feet. At ARM cord prolapse is more likely. In such cases, ARM should be delayed if the breech is not engaged and prostaglandin administered instead. If ARM is indicated it may be safer to carry this out in theatre where there is ready recourse to Caesarean section in the event of cord prolapse.

In the case of a footling presentation, ARM is contraindicated as the risk of cord prolapse either at amniotomy or later in labour is too great. An elective Caesarean section is the safer option.

Twin pregnancy

A significant proportion of multiple pregnancies will go into spontaneous labour preterm. Induction may be indicated because of associated PIH or because the pregnancy has advanced to 38 weeks. In the case of the latter it is generally considered safer to deliver rather than to await the spontaneous onset of labour, as the monitoring of fetal well-being becomes more difficult and there is increased risk of placental insufficiency. It is unusual for the cervix to be unfavourable so it is rarely necessary to 'ripen' with prostaglandins. Characteristically, labour in multiple pregnancy tends to be sluggish with a prolonged first stage. Syntocinon is usually required in addition to amniotomy to ensure adequate progress in labour.

If the first baby presents as a large breech or is other than a longitudinal lie, an elective Caesarean section will be the only safe method of delivery.

The presence of polyhydramnios can further complicate induction (see below).

Polyhydramnios

The chief risks arising from the induction of labour in the presence of polyhydramnios, are those associated with the sudden uncontrolled loss of amniotic fluid, and include:

- cord prolapse
- arm prolapse
- abruptio placentae
- sudden fetal distress.

When there is severe polyhydramnios, it is impossible to carry out a controlled fore-water rupture at ARM. No matter how the examining fingers are positioned, the liquor will gush over and between them and the operator will be unable to prevent a problem if it is going to occur. There are, therefore, three possible courses of action:

(1) decompress the uterus before ARM;
(2) ARM in the safest environment (theatre);
(3) elective Caesarean section.

When there is severe polyhydramnios, it is a relatively straightforward matter to carry out an amniocentesis under ultrasound control and remove 2–4 litres of liquor. This will considerably reduce the chances of a complication occuring at ARM. In less severe cases, to carry out the ARM in theatre at least means that the operator can rapidly cope with an emergency. This avoids the nightmare situation of trying to deal with such an emergency from a labour ward delivery room just as the registrar is starting a Caesarean section in theatre. There will always be situations where for fetal well-being it is preferable to deliver the baby by an elective Caesarean section.

Unstable lie

It is generally accepted that patients who present with an unstable lie from 38 weeks are admitted to hospital because of the risk of cord prolapse should spontaneous rupture of the membranes occur. At least being an in-patient at the time of such an event should increase the chance of the baby surviving. These patients are usually multiparous with a family to worry about and often resent just sitting on the ward waiting for something to happen. The reason for admission will have been explained, as well as the aim that, with luck, one or other pole of the baby will eventually enter the pelvic brim and so stabilize the lie, allowing an induction of labour to be safely performed. It is reasonable to point out that earlier intervention might result in an avoidable Caesarean section.

Repeated external versions are rather pointless when the lie is very unstable, as the baby will simply adopt a new lie. [Do not forget that the rhesus-negative patient requires to have anti-D immunoglobulin after version.]

Occasionally these pregnancies can be perverse and the lie remains unstable even when postmaturity threatens. In this situation, there is a place for considering a 'stabilizing induction'. On the labour ward, a medical induction is commenced either with a syntocinon infusion or vaginal PGE_2. By means of external version the lie is returned to the longitudinal with a cephalic presentation. (There is no place in modern obstetrics for using binders to try to maintain the lie as they do not work and are very uncomfortable.) The intention is that with the back-up of contractions the head will enter the pelvic brim and allow a later ARM to be carried out in safety. Should this not occur, Caesarean section remains the only alternative.

If polyhydramnios is the cause of the unstable lie, then amniocentesis as described above followed by a 'stabilizing induction' may succeed.

There will always be certain clinical situations when it will be considered preferable to deliver the baby via the abdominal route.

Previous Caesarean section (trial of scar)

A past history of a lower segment Caesarean section for a non-repetitive cause such as fetal distress or placenta praevia, is not in itself a contraindication to an induction of labour being carried out in the next pregnancy. If induction is indicated when the only previous delivery has been by Caesarean section, this is reasonable as long as there are no obvious contraindications such as cephalo-pelvic disproportion. When the patient has had an uneventful vaginal delivery of a term baby in a previous pregnancy, the pelvis has at least been 'proved' to be adequate. Induction should not present any problems when the cervix is 'favourable'.

The 'unfavourable' cervix, however, may present a problem if induction is indicated in the pregnancy following Caesarean section. The use of PGE_2 to 'ripen' the cervix can also have a similar effect upon the uterine scar with the dramatic consequences of a ruptured uterus. Under these circumstances, it may be considered to be preferable to deliver by means of an elective Caesarean section.

It is sometimes argued that neither syntocinon nor epidurals should be used when the previous delivery has been by Caesarean section owing to the increased risk of scar dehiscence. However, if a 'trial of scar' and vaginal delivery are being planned, then it is intended that contractions should occur every 2–3 minutes and last for 45 seconds. If syntocinon is required to achieve this aim, its use should not be contraindicated. Epidurals have been criticised for masking the pain of uterine scar rupture, but only 10 per cent of such cases actually feel pain. The more reliable signs of uterine rupture include:

- labour stops
- fetal distress → intrauterine death
- maternal tachycardia
- shock
- abnormal uterine contours (large broad ligament hamatomas)
- easily palpable fetal parts
- intrapartum bleeding.

Contraindications to a 'Trial of Scar'

- all the contraindications to induction (p. 139)
- a much larger baby
- all malpresentations
- multiple pregnancy
- intrauterine infection following Caesarean section
- tenderness over Caesarean scar.

If progress in labour is poor or complications arise, the 'trial of scar' is interrupted and the baby delivered by the speediest route.

Once full dilatation is reached, the 'trial of scar' is over. Rather than allow the additional stresses on the scar of the increased intrauterine pressures of the second stage of labour and maternal effort while pushing, the advantages of an elective forceps delivery should be considered.

After delivery, the lower segment should be assessed by an experienced clinician to determine whether or not the scar is intact. This is a straightforward procedure and a defect would be easily recognizable. Care must be taken not to actually perforate a scar by too vigorous an examination. If a small rupture is found, then this is noted and future deliveries will be by elective Caesarean section. A larger rupture, especially associated with bleeding, is an indication for laparotomy and repair of the scar site.

Intrauterine death (IUD)

Once an IUD has been diagnosed, it is only a kindness to the grieving couple to offer immediate admission with a view to the induction of labour. The majority of women find it abhorrent to have to await the spontaneous onset of labour. Great sensitivity, and indeed love, is required to help them over the hours ahead. Continuity of care by the midwifery team is extremely desirable. Obviously the only considerations must be for maternal safety and well-being.

A coagulation screen should be carried out before inducing labour to exclude any coagulopathy.

Induction of labour should not present any problem regardless of the gestational age of the fetus. **The induction *must* succeed**. Unless the cervix is very favourable, ARM and syntocinon will fail. The use of PGE$_2$ pessaries in the case of late IUD is generally successful in initiating the onset of labour. ARM and the subsequent synergistic effect of syntocinon will establish labour. In the case of earlier IUD the use of more potent prostaglandins in the form of gemeprost (Cervagem) pessaries may be indicated.

It is essential that adequate analgesia is available. To have to deliver a dead baby is distressing enough. At the very least, labour should be painless. This can either be achieved by epidural block or by the use of potent analgesics such as diamorphine 5 mg.

Very rarely an IUD can be complicated by a major degree of placenta praevia. Even in this difficult situation it should be possible to avoid Caesarean section. Delaying for a few days will result in a marked reduction in placental blood flow and allow a prostaglandin/syntocinon induction to be carried out. Blood should be cross-matched and readily available on the labour ward.

6   Labour and delivery

Although this may not be apparent to the woman and her partner, the labour ward must be regarded potentially as an intensive care area. Every pregnancy has the potential for producing a sudden and unexpected emergency.

> If a GP or midwife in the community is concerned about the well-being of an antenatal patient or her baby, then that patient should be seen promptly regardless of the time of day or night.

The labour ward is a useful 'sorting office', where, after initial assessment, a woman may be kept for closer observation or delivery, discharged home, or be sent to an antenatal ward for reassessment later.

> Every patient admitted to the labour ward of a consultant unit must be seen by a doctor for assessment.

The history and examination are essential features of this assessment. In the UK these will usually follow an initial assessment made by the admitting midwife who will have summarized the history and recorded the admission temperature, pulse, blood pressure, urine analysis, and the findings at abdominal examination. The abdominal palpation will determine the lie of the baby, the identification of the presenting part, whether or not it appears to be engaged in the pelvis, and the presence of a fetal heart. A CTG tracing is also helpful.

> A digital vaginal examination is contraindicated if the patient is not in labour and in cases of APH and premature rupture of membranes. IF IN DOUBT SEEK ADVICE.

Unless the patient is unbooked or has had no antenatal care, there are usually antenatal records available. Significant features of a previous delivery such as shoulder dystocia may be highlighted.

It may be very obvious that the patient is in established labour but this is not always the case. If she is experiencing contractions at least one in 10 minutes, has had a 'show', spontaneous rupture of membranes, or the cervix is found to be effaced and more than 3 cm dilated, then a diagnosis of labour is reasonable.

If the history suggests that the patient is in labour and there is no contraindication to carrying out a vaginal examination, then this is performed using an aseptic technique. All of the parameters used in determining the Bishop score are first assessed:

- dilatation of the cervix
- length of the cervix (effacement)
- consistency of the cervix
- position of the cervix
- station of the presenting part in relation to the ischial spines

then:

- identification of presenting part (cephalic or breech)
- position of presenting part
- degree of flexion
- degree of caput and moulding
- cervix well or poorly applied to presenting part
- membranes intact or ruptured
- appearance of liquor.

A clinical assessment of the adequacy of the pelvis is also made at this time.

All findings are recorded in the notes and the relevant details are entered onto a partogram. This gives a visual display of the progress of labour (Fig. 6.1).

If there is a query about management in labour NEVER HESITATE TO SEEK CONSULTANT ADVICE. This cannot be over-stressed.

A plan of management in labour may already have been decided upon. The woman's careplan should be considered and any reason to depart from this plan should be explained and discussed with her and her partner.

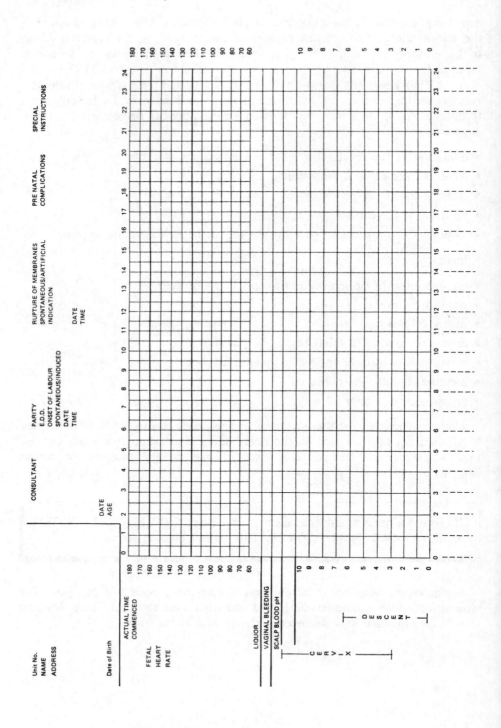

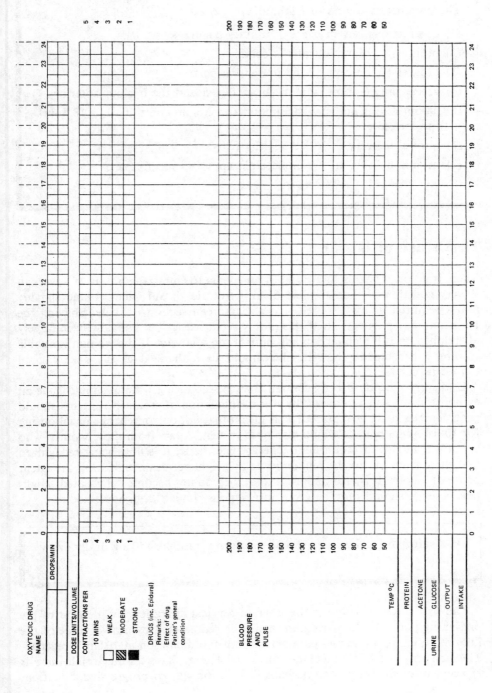

Fig. 6.1 Partogram.

The parameters for normal labour are:

(1) contractions one in every 3 minutes lasting 45 seconds;
(2) progressive dilatation of the cervix;
(3) progressive descent of the presenting part;
(4) vertex presentation with the bead flexed and the occiput anterior;
(5) labour lasting not less than 4 hours (precipitate) or more than 18 hours (prolonged);
(6) normal delivery of a live healthy baby;
(7) normal delivery of a complete placenta and membranes;
(8) NO COMPLICATIONS.

First stage of labour

There is no place for the old ritual of an enema to empty the bowel. If a woman is very constipated then the use of suppositories is sufficient. Pubic shaving is not required unless it is felt that a Caesarean section is likely. Shaving the perineum may make eventual episiotomy repair easier but has now been largely abandoned. A full bladder can add hours onto a labour. If the woman is unable to empty her bladder herself, she should be catherized at the next vaginal examination.

Until very recently it has been felt that the labouring woman should have an empty stomach so as to avoid the risk of inhalation of stomach contents should general anaesthesia be required. This meant that not only might she be labouring for 10–18 hours but she would also need to fast. Apart from those women who are at a high risk of requiring a general anaesthetic, it is now being recognized that there is no bar to the remainder taking light refreshment during the latent phase of labour. It is also important that they do not become dehydrated. High-risk patients should only be given intravenous fluids throughout labour.

As a safeguard, all women should be given ranitidine 150 mg orally every 6 hours.

The first stage of labour is the stage of cervical dilatation and descent of the presenting part. On the partogram it will be represented by a divergence of the lines representing these two parameters until full dilatation at 10 cm is reached. The first stage of labour includes an initial latent phase during which there is effacement of the cervix and perhaps little in the way of progressive dilatation.

During the active phase of labour, the cervix dilates at approximately 1 cm per hour for primiparous women and 2 cm per hour for multipara. A vaginal examination is carried out at least every 4 hours, **or more frequently if there is any concern about progress in labour.**

Regular assessments are made of:

- fetal heart rate quarter-hourly (Pinard or from CTG)
- maternal pulse rate half-hourly
- blood pressure half-hourly
- temperature 4-hourly
- urine analysis at each emptying of bladder

All examination findings are recorded onto the partogram.

Unless radio telemetry is employed, continuous fetal heart recording can only be performed if the woman is lying down. In the early hours of labour, especially if the membranes are still intact, it is reasonable for the woman to be mobile. If the membranes have ruptured, she should only be mobile if the presenting part is engaged in the pelvis and the cervix is well applied. Otherwise there is a risk of cord prolapse. When lying down, she should adopt whatever position she feels most comfortable in, whether on her side or reclining in a propped-up position. She should avoid lying flat on her back owing to the risks of supine hypotensive syndrome. Analgesia is provided when required (*see* pain relief, pp. 159–69).

If the patient is in labour with intact membranes and there are no obvious contraindications, ARM is indicated.

The advantages of ARM in labour

(1) increased efficiency of labour due to closer proximity of the presenting part to the cervix, thereby increasing the stimulus to labour;
(2) access to the fetus for fetal ECG and fetal blood sampling;
(3) permits observation of the appearance of meconium in the liquor.

If cervical dilatation increases by 2–4 cm between the first two vaginal examinations, no action needs to be taken. However, if cervical dilatation has not occurred, it may be necessary to augment labour with syntocinon.

> All patients who receive syntocinon to augment labour require continuous fetal heart monitoring.

Second stage of labour

This is the stage from full dilatation of the cervix to delivery of the baby. It is generally characterized by an overwhelming urge for the woman to push with her contractions. However, the urge to push may also occur late in the first stage, especially in multiparous patients. Confirmation of the second stage is obtained by finding that the cervix is fully dilated on vaginal examination or by seeing the fetal head without parting the labia.

For patients without an epidural, active pushing should not last more than one hour in primipara and half an hour in multipara. These times are not sacrosanct.

> If labour is progressing but taking a little longer, then this may be permitted as long as there is no concern for maternal or fetal well-being.

For those women who have an epidural, full dilatation is only likely to be diagnosed by vaginal examination. On the basis of the expected rate of dilatation for primipara and multipara, the probable time for full dilatation to be reached can be predicted and the vaginal examination can be timed accordingly. The finding of full dilatation under these circumstances does not mean that active maternal effort should commence unless the head is found to be on the perineum. It is perfectly reasonable to keep the epidural 'topped up' and allow further descent of the head over the next 2 hours. Continuous fetal heart monitoring is essential under these circumstances. When active pushing begins the epidural must not be allowed to 'wear off'. The contrast between being pain-free and experiencing the full pain of second-stage contractions can be devastating.

> The well-being of the mother and her baby remain paramount. Any cause for concern is an indication for intervention and rapid delivery.

When pushing commences, the woman should adopt whatever position suits her best. This is usually in a propped-up sitting position with several pillows or a wedge behind her. She should avoid lying flat on her back. She is encouraged to push with each contraction, drawing up her legs with a hand behind each knee. In between contractions she can rest.

To avoid confusion (and staff confrontation!) it is important that there is only one voice in command giving the woman instructions.

For a multiparous patient it is advisable for the person assisting the delivery to scrub up at this stage as occasionally only one or two pushes are required to complete the second stage.

Progress in the second stage can be determined by watching the vulval area. With descent of the head there is distension of the perianal veins whose venous return becomes obstructed. Gaping of the anus occurs as the perineum begins to bulge with further descent of the head. The occiput of the head is now just visible between the labia with each contraction. For a primiparous patient the assistant should scrub up at this point.

Extension of the head up the perineum now commences with each contraction, usually retreating a little after each push. Eventually the head remains distending the perineum and does not recede any further. (It is at this stage that it may be necessary to consider the need for an episiotomy.) The woman is warned that she should not push with the next contraction but pant rapidly. With the assistant standing on the woman's right side, the occiput is guarded with the left hand to prevent a sudden uncontrolled delivery of the head while a pad is held over the anus. The head is delivered in between contractions by applying pressure with the pad beneath the fetal chin to encourage further extension and so allows the perineum to sweep over the face and chin. During this time the woman is instructed not to push but to pant rapidly so that she actually breathes out the delivery of the head rather than actively pushes.

The baby's face is cleaned and mucus is aspirated from the mouth, nose, and pharynx. The assistant feels around the baby's neck for a loop of cord. If the cord is felt it can either be lifted over the baby's head or divided between Spencer–Wells forceps. There is now restitution of the baby's head on the neck into an occipito-lateral position as the shoulders rotate to take up an antero-posterior position prior to delivery of the anterior shoulder.

With the next contraction, the patient is asked to push once again. The assistant draws the head down towards the anus and so delivers the anterior shoulder beneath the pubic arch. At this point the woman is given an intramuscular injection of syntometrine containing 5 units of syntocinon and 0.5 mg of ergometrine. The head is then drawn up towards the symphysis and the posterior shoulder emerges above the perineum. The baby is then delivered across the woman's abdomen. If not already divided the cord is clamped with a plastic umbilical clip. The baby is wrapped up in a warm blanket and handed over to its mother.

Third stage of labour

This is the interval between the delivery of the baby and the delivery of the placenta. It is a potentially hazardous time because of the risks of postpartum haemorrhage. Vigilance can also be a little relaxed in the general euphoria associated with a successful delivery.

Placental separation usually occurs within a few minutes of delivery. In the bustle associated with wrapping up the baby and general tidying up in readiness for the delivery of the placenta, the signs of separation may be missed. These include:

- the fundus of the uterus rises in the abdomen
- lengthening of the cord
- a show of blood (which could also be the beginning of a postpartum haemorrhage!)

In modern obstetric practice the third stage is actively managed, but when problems do occur they are usually associated with too speedy an attempt to achieve delivery of the placenta.

The principles of third stage management

1. Look for the signs of placental separation.
2. NEVER attempt to deliver the placenta unless the uterus is well contracted

The delivery assistant remains on the woman's right side after delivery of the baby. The uterus is confirmed to be well contracted. The cord clamp is shifted so as to be positioned on the cord at the vulva. The assistant then places the left hand firmly above the symphysis and applies gentle pressure towards the maternal back but also in an upward direction. This movement firstly aligns the uterus with the long axis of the vagina to facilitate delivery when cord traction is applied and secondly will prevent any tendency of the fundus of the uterus to invert and 'follow' the placenta into the vagina.

While maintaining the direction of pressure with the left hand, the right hand applies *gentle* cord traction downwards towards the bed at an angle of about 45 degrees from the horizontal plane. The tensile strength of the cord is such that it can sustain a pressure of up to 3.5 kg before rupturing.

As the placenta descends, the angle of traction on the cord becomes more horizontal. As the placenta 'climbs the perineum' the angle of traction is raised to 45 degrees above the horizontal plane.

During the actual delivery of the placenta cord traction ceases. The right hand takes the weight of the placenta while also rotating it so as to wind the membranes into a rope. This action controls the speed of delivery of the placenta and increases the likelihood that the membranes will be delivered completely.

> During controlled cord traction, the left hand is not removed from its suprapubic position until the delivery of the placenta is completed.

If the placenta does not seem to be descending, do not increase the strength of traction. This will only increase the probability of the cord rupturing and the subsequent need for a manual removal of the placenta. It may be that separation of the placenta has not yet occurred and the active management has simply been premature.

1. Wait.
2. Is the bladder empty?
3. Is the cervix clamped around the placenta?
4. Use maternal effort to assist in the delivery.
5. If the placenta is not delivered within 20 minutes, seek help.

> There is a strange reluctance to perform a vaginal examination during the third stage of labour. It can be most informative.

The placenta, cord, and membranes must be inspected carefully for completeness and for any abnormalities.

> If in doubt, SEEK ADVICE.

Pain relief in labour

Many women will have indicated their preferences for a particular form of pain relief in labour while drawing up their careplans. As far as possible these wishes should be complied with and any indication to depart from the plan fully discussed. A significant proportion of women, especially primigravidae, regard labour with dread. One of the major roles of antenatal care is to inform and educate and, as far as possible, remove fear which is often based upon ignorance. It is also important to allay any feelings of guilt should the woman subsequently change her mind in labour and choose complete analgesia. Even for those women who do not wish to opt for the prospect of complete analgesia which a regional block should provide, the knowledge that such a service is available if required, can be very reassuring. In contrast, some women will only be able to contemplate the possibility of labouring if they can be certain of receiving total analgesia. A sympathetic consultant obstetric anaesthetist therefore plays an important role in discussing the pain relief services available during antenatal classes.

Familiarity with the labour ward suite by guided tour can remove some of the fear of the unknown. Obviously pleasant surroundings, the comforts of a 'home-from-home unit', and the availability of music can do much create a supportive atmosphere.

Options for pain relief in labour

Non-pharmacological:
  psychoprophylaxis
  water birth
  transdermal electrical nerve stimulation

Opiate analgesia

Inhalation analgesia

Local anaesthesia:
  perineal infilitration
  pudendal block
  epidural block
  spinal block

General anaesthesia

Non-pharmacological pain relief

Psychoprophylaxis

Antenatally both the woman and her partner will have attended classes where everything possible is done to reduce fear and to inform the couple of what can be expected in labour. They will have been jointly trained in techniques which amount to distraction therapy. The involvement and support of the woman's partner is essential for the success of this method, as is the understanding of the midwives attending the patient. In labours that are short and efficient, especially for multiparous women, psychoprophylaxis may enable the patient to cope without any other form of pain relief. In longer labours additional analgesia is often required. It is under these circumstances that feelings of guilt over having 'let myself down' or having 'let my partner down' are likely to arise. The attending midwife has a very important role to ensure that this does not occur.

Water births

Many women who experience delivery in a birthing pool claim significant pain relief from the relaxation, mobility, and weightlessness that is achieved. Usually, if additional analgesia is required, inhalation analgesia with Entonox is sufficient. However, electronic fetal monitoring cannot be performed under water. There is also concern regarding the risks of infection and the apparent increase in the incidence of primary postpartum haemorrhage as well as tragic cases of fetal mortality. While it is acknowledged that to be immersed in warm water may be very soothing during the first stage of labour, it is quite another matter to deliver the baby in this environment. Those women who state that they will leave the pool at the end of the first stage may find it a physically impossible feat to achieve. Most birthing pools have steep sides and seem to be poorly designed for rapid patient transfer. Midwives who wish to be involved in water births must be adequately trained and not 'learn as they go'. Controlled trials are essential to fully evaluate the benefits of water births.

Transdermal electrical nerve stimulation (TENS)

TENS involves the use of low-level, pulsed, electrical currents via surface electrodes which are placed upon the skin of the back. The level of stimulation is totally controlled by the patient and can be effective in blocking some of the pain that would otherwise be experienced in early labour. The woman adjusts the strength of pulses to the highest level she finds is comfortable. It is also possible to boost the pulse rate during contractions. The effect is similar to that produced by rubbing the back and sacrum and so stimulating an area of referred pain. This may involve the release of endorphins which reduce the awareness of pain. It is ideal in short labours and is often used in conjunction with inhalation analgesia in the second stage of labour. It is totally non-invasive and has no known side effects. The only contraindication to its use is the patient who has a cardiac pacemaker. TENS kits can be hired in the UK for 4-week periods from the manufacturing company.

Opiate analgesia

The commonest opiate analgesic that is used in the UK during the first stage of labour is **pethidine**. To be effective, this is administered in a dosage of 100–150 mg intramuscularly on a 4-hourly basis. Ideally, pethidine should be avoided during the 4 hours prior to delivery because of the mild respiratory depressant effect that it has on the newborn baby, but this timing can be difficult to judge. However, fear of the proximity of delivery should not prevent the use of pethidine, as naloxone is a specific antagonist should there be evidence of respiratory depression.

Pethidine requires 20 minutes to become effective when given via the intramuscular route. For up to 40 per cent of patients the degree of pain relief is inadequate. Rapid pain relief can be achieved by giving 25 mg intravenously. If available, PCAS (patient-controlled analgesia system) will deliver a bolus of pethidine 10 mg intravenously whenever the patient feels it is required. PCAS utilizes a 10-minute 'lock out' after each bolus so that excess analgesia cannot be given.

If nausea is a marked side-effect, prochlorperazine (Stemetil) 12.5 mg intramuscularly is very effective.

There is a place for the use of stronger opiates such as **morphine** 10 mg and **diamorphine** 5 mg intravenously. For those prolonged labours where epidurals are not available, it is perfectly justifiable to use these preparations. The respiratory depression effect on the fetus is greater but may be reversed with naloxone. There is also a place for using these drugs where the well-being of the baby does not arise, as in the case of gross fetal abnormality and intrauterine death.

Opiates must not be used if there has been a known hypersensitivity reaction in the past, a history of narcotic abuse, or if currently using monoamine oxidase inhibitors.

Inhalation analgesia

The place for inhalation analgesia is late in the first stage when the woman is being asked not to push in spite of an often overwhelming urge to do so, and during the second stage of labour. **Entonox** (nitrous oxide 50 per cent and oxygen 50 per cent) is ideal for this purpose. It is self-administered by the woman, who should have received instruction in its use antenatally. Entonox should be inhaled as soon as a contraction is perceived, whether by the CTG or on palpation, but before pain is experienced. The patient is instructed to inhale deeply via the face mask or mouthpiece so that the Entonox apparatus makes a clicking sound, indicating release of the gas. She should exhale rapidly before taking another deep breath.

Entonox has a rapid analgesic effect within 15–20 seconds of inhalation. There is no risk of cumulative effects on the patient and no respiratory depressive effect on the baby. It is expelled very rapidly from the body and can therefore be used for long periods of time. If the woman shows signs of becoming anaesthetized she will simply stop inhaling with the force required to trigger the release of more Entonox and will rapidly recover.

During the second stage of labour, the patient should be instructed to use the Entonox continuously and to take two or three quick breaths of gas before each push.

DON'T LET THE ENTONOX CYLINDER RUN OUT! This will cause acute panic!

Local anaesthesia

Perineal infiltration

The commonest indication for the perineal infiltration of a local anaesthetic is episiotomy (p. 179). Episiotomy is something which a woman may be more terrified over than the actual birth process. She may have heard reports of painful experiences from other women and specifically request that no episiotomy should be carried out when completing her careplan. One of the roles of antenatal care is to remove fear, especially when linked to lack of knowledge about the subject. The fact that episiotomy is sometimes necessary should be explained antenatally and assurance given that the actual procedure should be relatively painless.

> Even in an emergency situation there is ALWAYS time to infiltrate with local anaesthetic before episiotomy.

The most commonly used local anaesthetic agent is lignocaine (Xylocaine). The maximum recommended dosage of lignocaine is 200 mg (1 ml of 1% lignocaine is equivalent to 10 mg lignocaine). Side-effects are uncommon unless the maximum dosage has been considerably exceeded, or the lignocaine has inadvertently been given intravenously. If it is invisaged that much larger volumes than 20 ml will be required, it is safer (and just as effective) to use a 0.5 per cent strength of lignocaine.

> To avoid accidental intravenous injection, always draw back on the syringe before infiltration to ensure that the needle is not in a vessel.

Preparations containing lignocaine and adrenaline should be avoided. Side-effects include rare drug idiosyncrasy or hypersensitivity and rare systemic effects involving the central nervous system and cardiovascular system. Good anaesthesia is usually achieved within 5 minutes and should have a duration of 30–45 minutes.

It is first explained that the area is going to be 'numbed' with a local anaesthetic. Using an aseptic technique, two fingers are inserted into the vagina to protect the fetus from needle injury. Ten to 20 ml of lignocaine 0.5–1% (without adrenaline) is infiltrated fanwise from the mid-point of the fourchette. This should be done with a single skin puncture as the direction of the needle can easily be changed without complete withdrawal. The superficial subcutaneous tissues over the planned episiotomy site are first infiltrated before repeating the process for the deeper parts of the perineum. It is also advantageous to inject a few millilitres of lignocaine into the lower margins of each labium minus.

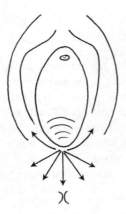

Fig. 6.2   Perineal infiltration.

Perineal infiltration as described may provide adequate analgesia for low 'lift-out' forceps deliveries where the head is resting on the perineum. It is also often carried out to supplement a pudendal block.

Pudendal block

Pudendal block is indicated for pelvic manipulative procedures including mid-cavity and low forceps, ventouse, and rotational forceps deliveries. If it is known that the procedure is going to be difficult, a pudendal block may not be the appropriate form of analgesia. The target of a pudendal block is each pudendal nerve (S. 2, 3, 4) with additional perineal infiltration blocking fibres of S. 5. It can be seen that a pudendal block would not be suitable for uterine surgery as higher sensory nerve roots would need to be blocked.

The planned procedure is explained to the woman. She is placed into the lithotomy position, and the vulva and perineum are cleaned and draped. The bladder is emptied. A vaginal examination is performed gently. Depending upon the degree of discomfort the patient is experiencing, it may be preferable to carry out a perineal infiltration at this stage rather than after the pudendal block has been given. Entonox may be used during the administration of the block.

Firstly 20 ml of 1% lignocaine are drawn up into a syringe which is attached to a transvaginal pudendal block needle. A vaginal examination is performed with two fingers of the right hand and the right ischial spine is located. An outer pudendal needle guide is passed between the two examining fingers so that the bulbous tip of the guide is pressing just below the ischial spine. Some forms of the guide have a proximal ring for the thumb of the examining hand. The pudendal needle with the syringe attached is then introduced into the needle guide. As the pudendal needle is longer than the outer guide, it will be inserted into the area below and behind the ischial spine. Before injecting any lignocaine, the needle is aspirated to ensure that it has not entered a blood vessel. If blood should be drawn back into the syringe the needle is resited; 10 ml of lignocaine is then injected at this site. The procedure is repeated on the opposite side.

Epidural block

Epidural blocks are the ideal form of analgesia in obstetric practice as total pain relief can be obtained.

Indications for epidural block

- patient request
- inadequate opiate or inhalation analgesia
- hypertensive disorders
- in anticipation of instrumental delivery
- prolonged labour
- maternal distress/exhaustion
- preterm labour
- trial of labour
- multiple pregnancy
- elective Caesarean section.

Epidurals may be given via the lumbar or caudal route and there are advantages and disadvantages to both. Generally the lumbar route is preferred for its speed of action and more certain success rate, although caudal blocks provide better pelvic and perineal analgesia and are unlikely to result in an accidental dural tap.

The procedure should be explained to the woman, informing her particularly about the loss of sensation she will experience over the abdomen and legs and the variable degree of motor paralysis that can occur while the block is effective. She should be told that she may find it more difficult to push in the second stage of labour as she will not feel her contractions. Her consent is obtained.

It is essential that experienced staff are constantly available, both to perform the epidural and subsequently to monitor the patient.

Because of the risks of hypotension following an epidural, it is essential that an intravenous infusion of Hartmann's solution is set up before the epidural block is commenced. The woman is positioned either sitting forwards and supported on the edge of the bed or in a left lateral position with her head and knees tucked in. Both of these positions will have the effect of opening up the intervertebral spaces as much as possible. Remember that it can be extremely difficult for the patient in strong labour to remain still, which is vital at the precise time that the epidural needle is inserted. There is, therefore, some advantage in siting an epidural in early labour so that it is available for later use when labour is more fully established.

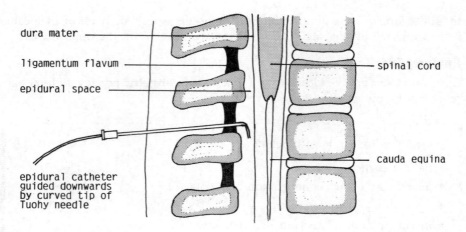

Fig. 6.3   Epidural block.

The skin over the lumbar area of the back is cleaned and draped. Lignocaine 0.5–1% is infiltrated into the desired intervertebral space between L3 and L5. A Tuohy needle is passed through the skin and ligamentum flavum. The epidural space is recognized by using a 'loss of resistance' technique from an air-filled syringe attached to the needle. As the needle is advanced, the syringe plunger suddenly 'gives' as the epidural space is entered.

An epidural catheter is then passed along the Tuohy needle, the curved tip of which directs the catheter downwards into the epidural space. The needle is then withdrawn over the catheter which is left *in situ*. Great care is now taken to ensure that no blood or cerebrospinal fluid (CSF) is seen leaking back along the catheter. If blood is seen, it is probable that the catheter has been introduced into a vein. The catheter is withdrawn and the epidural is resited. If CSF is seen, a diagnosis of dural tap is made. The catheter must be withdrawn and the epidural resited. The epidural puncture site is sprayed with an antiseptic and the catheter is firmly strapped to the patient's back and led up to her shoulder. A bacterial filter is attached to the catheter.

Failure to recognize a dural tap and proceeding with the epidural block can lead to the serious complication of an accidental full spinal anaesthetic, resulting in profound hypotension and respiratory arrest. It is, therefore, vital that staff capable of resuscitation and intubation are constantly available.

As a further precaution, a test dose must always be given before the full epidural is administered. Two millilitres of lignocaine 2% is a standard test dose. The blood pressure is checked every 5 minutes over the next 10 minutes. It is safe to proceed with the full epidural if there is no sign of the test dose having produced analgesia.

The longer-acting local anaesthetic bupivacaine (Marcaine) 0.25, 0.375 or 0.5% is the preparation most commonly used to produce an epidural block.

After the full epidural dosage has been given, the patient is closely monitored with blood pressure checks every 5 minutes for the first 20 minutes and then half-hourly checks. The patient is nursed on her side and then turned to get even distribution of the block. A partial block is not uncommon. If this occurs, the patient lies on the unblocked side while a further dose of anaesthetic is given. Occasionally the catheter will require to be withdrawn slightly to correct the problem.

> Continuous fetal heart monitoring is essential during and after epidural block.

When 'top-ups' are required, these may be given by suitably trained mid-wifery staff. The timing and dosage of the 'top-ups' will be determined by the anaesthetist.

In the event of a dural tap, the patient must be kept in a restful state through out labour. She is given Hartmann's solution one litre intravenously every 6 hours. She will not be allowed to push in the second stage, but instead is delivered by elective forceps to reduce further leakage of CSF. Severe headaches are common after dural tap and can persist for several days. The best treatment is to administer a postnatal epidural infusion of one litre of normal saline 12-hourly for 24 hours via the bacterial filter. If this should fail to relieve severe symptoms, an epidural 'blood patch' should be carried out by the anaesthetist.

Disadvantages of epidural block
Total analgesia can present a problem in the second stage of labour. There may be no sensation at all of even strong contractions so there is no urge to push. As a result it is perfectly reasonable to allow another 2 hours for the head to descend further before maternal effort is attempted. The fetal heart must be continuously monitored during this time. Any concern for fetal well-being will indicate a need for immediate forceps delivery.

Similarly, it can be difficult for the woman to empty her bladder and she may require intermittent catheterization.

The situation will frequently arise, that a patient with a successful epidural block will require a non-emergency Caesarean section. This does not present a problem as very satisfactory anaesthesia can be achieved and the epidural can be used for postoperative analgesia. However, if an emergency arises indicating a need for very urgent delivery, the epidural block will not permit the operator to employ the same degree of speed that can be used under general anaesthesia. Under such circumstances, a general anaesthetic in addition to the epidural is preferable. It is worth while mentioning this possibility to every woman receiving an epidural block in labour so as to avoid major disappointment if a sudden emergency arises.

An epidural Caesarean section is a moving and notable experience for many couples. Together, they can experience the most dramatic form of entry of their baby into their lives. Note that this is not the right environment for a junior registrar to be seen to be receiving training in how to carry out a Caesarean section! Expertise, calmness, and gentleness are absolute requirements for epidural surgery.

Contraindications to epidural block

(1) inadequate facilities/experience to look after the patient;

(2) patient refusal;

(3) infection at planned epidural site;

(4) coagulopathy: severe PIH and abruptio placentae → disseminated intravascular coagulopathy;

(5) anticoagulant therapy;

(6) major lumbar disc problems;

(7) chronic neurological disease;

(8) a need for speed at Caesarean section;

(9) elective Caesarean section for an anterior placenta praevia.

Spinal block

A spinal (subarachnoid) block is a useful method of achieving anaesthesia when speed is required. It is generally given as a 'single-shot' injection to provide anaesthesia for a short procedure such as a forceps delivery or the manual removal of a retained placenta. With the patient in a sitting position, 1.5 ml of bupivocaine 0.5% is injected into the subarachnoid space at the level of L. 3–4. Spinal block can rapidly provide sufficient anaesthesia to carry out Caesarean section, especially for the patient who is not suitable for general anaesthesia.

General anaesthesia

Obstetric emergencies demanding rapid surgical intervention are an everyday feature of a busy labour ward. The great advantage of general anaesthesia over epidural block is speed. The attendant risks of emergency anaesthesia are therefore significantly greater than for cold elective surgery.

In the UK there has been a significant reduction in the number of maternal deaths either directly due to or associated with obstetric anaesthesia. This is due to an increase in obstetric anaesthesia resources, increased awareness of the risks of obstetric anaesthesia, and the greater use of epidural anaesthesia. However, general anaesthesia still features as a cause of maternal death. The major causes of death directly due to general anaesthesia include:

(1) endotracheal tube problems;

(2) aspiration of gastric contents → Mendelson's syndrome;

(3) inadequate monitoring during surgery;

(4) failure of postoperative care.

Inappropriate delegation of obstetric anaesthesia to inexperienced anaesthetists, the lack of trained anaesthetic assistants, the lack of fully-equipped, designated recovery areas with nursing staff trained in the care of the unconscious patient, the lack of high-dependency care areas that are equipped for resuscitation and respiratory and cardiovascular monitoring, and poor communication between obstetrician and anaesthetist over potential anaesthetic problems are all implicated in the Confidential Enquiries into Maternal Deaths in the UK.

While it has been normal practice to starve all women undergoing elective Caesarean section, there is evidence that this actually increases the acidity of gastric contents. The gastric contents of the labouring patient who suddenly requires emergency surgery will be very variable. Every patient on the labour ward should, therefore, be regarded as a potential candidate for emergency surgery.

To effectively reduce the production of acidic gastric contents, all patients in labour should receive the H_2-receptor blocker **ranitidine** 150 mg orally 6-hourly. Many units will also use 20–30 ml of 0.3 M sodium citrate orally, to be given when the decision to operate is made and then repeated upon arrival in the anaesthetic room if a general anaesthetic is to be given.

The other risk of starvation is dehydration. Unless delivery is imminent, intravenous fluids should be given after 6 hours of starvation. One litre of 5% dextrose in half-strength Hartmann's solution is given in 12 hours.

Once on the operating table, the patient is tilted laterally towards the side of the operator to prevent supine hypotension. Prior to the induction of anaesthesia, pre-oxygenation with 100 per cent oxygen is carried out for several minutes to reduce fetal hypoxia. The obstetrician should clean and drape the abdomen during this time so as to reduce fetal exposure to anaesthetic agents. The anaesthetist will explain to the woman the sensation she will experience when cricoid pressure is applied. Anaesthesia is induced with intravenous thiopentone and cricoid pressure is applied by the anaesthetic assistant. A muscle relaxant is given to allow a cuffed endotracheal intubation to be introduced. Only when the cuff is inflated is the cricoid pressure released. Nitrous oxide and oxygen maintain the anaesthetic.

Operative awareness by the patient is the risk of light obstetric anaesthesia. The anaesthetist must ensure that the depth of anaesthesia is sufficient to prevent this terrifying experience.

Fetal monitoring during labour

The assessment of fetal well-being is one of the major aims of antenatal care and is only concluded by the delivery of the baby. Labour is potentially the most dangerous environment for every fetus, as the placenta and its ability to maintain fetal oxygenation are being stressed with every contraction. Fetal distress in labour can be insidious and difficult to diagnose, or dramatic and short-lived. Its early detection is imperative. Intrauterine death in labour which has been preceded by clear signs of fetal distress is indefensible.

Methods used to monitor fetal well-being in labour:

(1) fetal heart rate monitoring:
    auscultation
    cardiotocography;
(2) observation of liquor to detect meconium;
(3) fetal blood sampling.

Fetal heart rate monitoring

During an uncomplicated first stage of labour, quarter-hourly recordings of the fetal heart rate using a Pinard fetal stethoscope are perfectly adequate. During the second stage of labour, the heart rate should be listened to after each contraction. When labour is being induced, augmented, an epidural block is used for pain relief, or the pregnancy is considered to be at 'high risk', continuous fetal heart rate monitoring by cardiotocography is indicated.

The normal fetal heart rate in labour ranges between 120 and 160 beats per minute. When using a Pinard fetal stethoscope, it is usually impossible to hear the fetal heart during a strong contraction. The ideal time to determine the fetal heart rate is immediately after a contraction, as this will then pick up any late decelerations of the fetal heart. A portable, ultrasound, fetal heart detector can be used to confirm any heart rate irregularities, which would then indicate the need for continuous heart rate monitoring.

Cardiotocography (CTG) is used routinely as a means of monitoring fetal well-being antenatally (p. 29). In labour, CTG permits continuous fetal heart monitoring up to the point of delivery. Whereas the antenatal CTG must employ an external ultrasound transducer, in labour either the external transducer or a fetal ECG can be used. In the latter, a clip is attached to either the scalp or the breech of the baby. The major advantages that the fetal ECG has over the external transducer are that usually the quality of tracing obtained is superior and there is no loss of contact which interrupts the trace when the baby moves.

The features of the normal CTG in labour are the same as for the antenatal tracing and include:

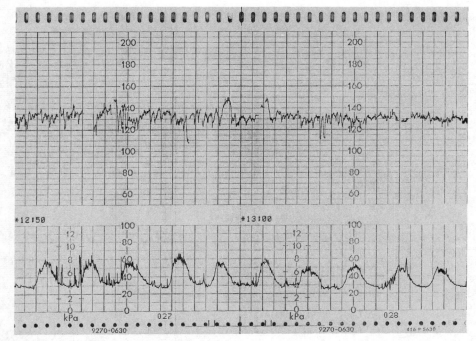

Fig. 6.4   Normal CTG in labour.

- baseline rate of 120–160 per minute
- variability greater than five beats per minute
- accelerations of the fetal heart during contractions
- no decelerations
- contractions of the uterus.

(See Fig. 6.4.)

Uncomplicated moderate bradycardias or tachycardias beyond the 120–160 limits need not in themselves cause concern, as long as the variability is satisfactory and there are no decelerations (Fig. 6.5 and 6.6).

Variability may be reduced as a result of opiates or sedation.

A *complete* loss of variability indicates a grim prognosis. **Urgent delivery is essential**.

See Fig. 6.7.

Decelerations that mirror the contractions and return to the baseline when the contraction ceases do not imply fetal distress, as long as there is good variability.

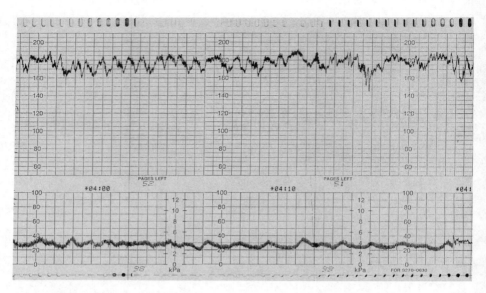

Fig. 6.5 Uncomplicated tachycardia in labour.

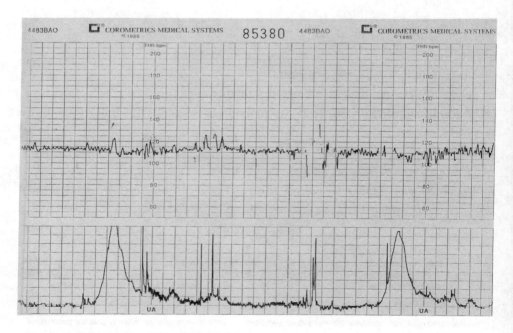

Fig. 6.6 Baseline bradycardia in labour.

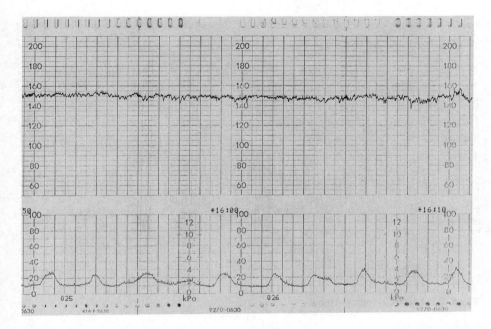

Fig. 6.7   Flat CTG in labour, followed by severe fetal distress, leading to emergency Caesarean section.

These Type I decelerations are usually due to compression of the fetal head during contractions (Fig. 6.8).

Type I decelerations that are very variable in either timing or shape may indicate cord compression which could compromise the fetus (Fig. 6.9).

Delay in the recovery of a deceleration to the normal baseline is more worrying and indicates a need for fetal blood sampling (Fig. 6.10).

Late (Type II) decelerations which commence before the contraction is completed and persist after the stress of the contraction is gone must always be regarded seriously (Fig. 6.11).

In the first stage of labour, ANY CTG that causes worry is *at least* an indication for fetal blood sampling.

There will always be situations where merely a worry will be an indication for operative delivery. For example, the patient who has a grim past obstetric history with no living children should, if the CTG is worrying, be delivered by Caesarean section.

The CTG becomes more difficult to interpret during the second stage of labour, especially when maternal effort is actively employed. However the

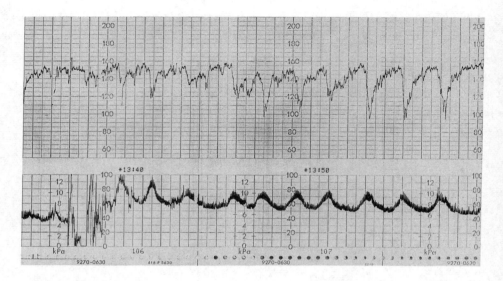

Fig. 6.8   Type I decelerations.

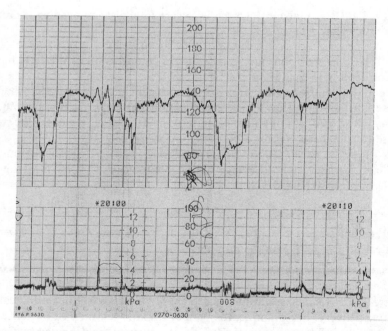

Fig. 6.9   Variable decelerations typical of cord compression. FBS pH 7.33, slight meconium; 2 hours later FBS 7.28 at 3 cm dilation. At 5 cm, prolonged deceleration. Emergency Caesarean section.

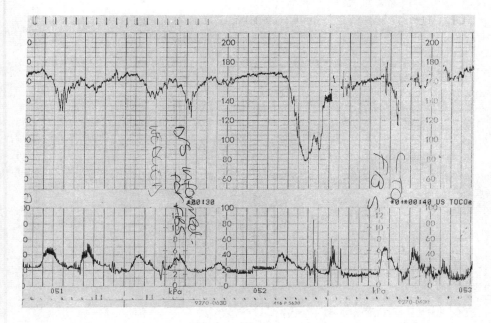

Fig. 6.10   Late deceleration. FBS 7.19, emergency Caesarean section. Apgar 3 + 7.

cardinal rules regarding a normal CTG still apply. Loss of variability and/or major decelerations indicate that delivery is urgent.

> There is no place for fetal blood sampling in the second stage of labour. Get the baby delivered!

Observation of liquor to detect meconium

In order to be able to observe the liquor in labour, the membranes must be ruptured. If the membranes are ruptured late in labour and meconium staining of the liquor is noted, it is impossible to know the length of time the meconium has been present. However, if amniotomy is performed early in labour and the liquor is initially clear, the subsequent appearance of meconium may be very significant.

The presence of meconium in the amniotic fluid does not in itself necessarily imply fetal hypoxia. Conversely, the absence of meconium cannot give reassurance that all is well, as a proportion of stillborn infants never pass meconium. If the liquor volume is scanty, meconium may not be seen, even if it is passed.

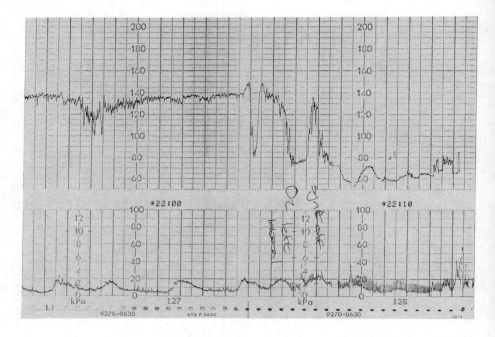

Fig. 6.11 Sudden deceleration at 9 cm. Ventouse delivery. Apgar 9 + 9.

If the fetal head is deeply engaged and the cervix well applied, meconium may be trapped in the liquor behind the head and only be revealed at delivery.

Because hypoxia can cause the fetus to relax its anal sphincter, the presence of meconium staining in the liquor is an indication for continuous fetal heart rate monitoring by CTG. If any abnormal CTG patterns develop, fetal blood sampling is carried out.

Occasionally very heavy 'pea soup' thick, fresh meconium is found. This is invariably associated with hypoxia and is an indication for urgent delivery.

A paediatrician should always be present at delivery when meconium is present. Meconium aspiration by the baby can have a poor outcome. Aspiration of meconium from the trachea and bronchi on delivery may prevent a fatal pneumonia.

Fetal blood sampling (FBS)

The normal fetal pH is 7.3 ± 0.05. When the fetus becomes hypoxic, there is a build-up of lactic acid leading to fetal acidosis and a lowering of the fetal pH. The fetal hypoxia will lead to changes in the fetal heart rate. Fetal blood sampling permits a more accurate assessment of fetal well-being.

Indications for fetal blood sampling are

- a worrying CTG
- meconium in the liquor
- an earlier borderline FBS.

Before carrying out an FBS, the current situation should be discussed with the woman, and the need for sampling explained. She should be reassured that taking an FBS will not cause distress or harm to the baby.

She is either placed into lithotomy (with a wedge to bring about 15 degrees of tilt to prevent supine hypotension) or into a left lateral position. The perineal area is cleaned and draped. Using an aseptic technique, a vaginal examination is performed to assess the degree of cervical dilatation. As long as the cervix is at least 3 cm dilated, an amnioscope of the appropriate diameter is guided by the examining fingers through the cervix, ensuring that no cervix is trapped between the amnioscope and fetal scalp (or buttock). A light source is fitted to the amnioscope. Maintaining close contact between the amnioscope and fetal scalp to prevent the leakage of liquor into the amnioscope, the scalp is cleaned and dried. An assistant sprays the scalp with ethyl chloride as the reactive hyperaemia which follows improves the prospects of obtaining a satisfactory FBS. Silicone jelly is then applied to the scalp as this will encourage the blood released at sampling to form a globule and so facilitate collection. Using a special 2 mm guarded blade, a single stab is made into the fetal scalp. Occasionally a second stab is required. The tip of a heparinized glass collection tube is placed in contact with the blood globule without touching the scalp. It is usually possible to collect the sample by gravitation but sometimes very gentle suction is necessary. The aim is to collect an uninterrupted column of blood into the tube. Haemostasis is achieved by applying pressure with a small swab against the stab site. Meanwhile, as the sample is taken to the pH meter, it is mixed in the tube by introducing a tiny metal rod which is moved through the blood column using an external magnet.

Interpretation of FBS pH results

- pH > 7.25 is normal
- pH 7.2–7.25 is borderline and should be repeated within 30 minutes
- pH < 7.20 indicates significant acidosis and a need for urgent delivery to avoid fetal death.

Diagnosis of fetal distress

In the past, the diagnosis of fetal distress was based upon abnormalities of the fetal heart rate at auscultation and/or the appearance of meconium in the liquor. As a result, a significant number of unnecessary Caesarean sections will have been performed. Continuous fetal heart rate monitoring has made it possible to detect the CTG features which indicate a need for further action by FBS or intervention by delivery.

An additional feature that is occasionally noted by the woman who presents with an intrauterine death, is that the last movements that the baby made were very excessive, as if the baby was trying 'to fight its way out'. If this is noted in labour, further intensive monitoring by CTG and FBS is vital.

When there is an indication to deliver urgently, then urgency is exactly what is required.

When fetal distress occurs during the first stage of labour, the only option is to deliver the baby by emergency Caesarean section, preferably under general anaesthesia.

Even with a functioning epidural block, Caesarean section under additional general anaesthesia permits maximum speed.

During the second stage of labour, the options for delivery are via either the vaginal or abdominal routes. Sometimes an episiotomy performed when the patient is in lithotomy, in readiness for a forceps delivery, is all that is required. Forceps deliveries, including rotational deliveries, are preferable to using the ventouse. However, fetal distress at any stage in labour in a breech presentation is an indication for emergency Caesarean section.

REMEMBER that a vaginal delivery may not always be the best option if considerable difficulty can be foreseen.

Episiotomy and perineal tears

Episiotomy

Episiotomy is an operative procedure to enlarge the introitus of the vagina at delivery. It should never be carried out as a routine procedure.

Indications for episiotomy

(1) fetal distress with the head on the perineum;

(2) an unyielding perineum delaying delivery of the head;

(3) forceps deliveries;

(4) breech deliveries;

(5) delivery of a preterm baby;

(6) previous third-degree tear;

(7) perineal tear is imminent, particularly for 'buttonholing' of a thinned-out perineum.

There is always time to anaesthetize the perineum (p. 163) even in the most extreme emergency. Cutting through the unanaesthetized perineum 'at the height of a contraction' is barbaric.

The timing of an episiotomy is important and takes considerable skill and experience. If it is carried out too early, it achieves nothing and the cut edges can bleed profusely. The correct time is when the perineum is distended by the presenting part. During the infiltration of local anaesthetic and then during the episiotomy, two fingers of the left hand are inserted inside the vagina between the fourchette and the presenting part of the baby to protect the baby from injury by, firstly, the needle and, secondly, the scissors. A sharp pair of scissors is the best instrument with which to perform an episiotomy. The scissors are opened and one blade is inserted into the vagina between the internal fingers and fourchette. The cut should start from the mid-point of the fourchette and pass initially downwards towards the anus. The scissors are then angled to convert the incision into a 'J' shape with the lower half of the episiotomy directed approximately 1 cm lateral to the anal margin (Fig. 6.12).

The medio-lateral episiotomy also starts at the mid-point of the fourchette and is directed towards the ischial tuberosity. As more muscle is cut than for a 'J'-shaped episiotomy, potentially more bruising and discomfort may occur postnatally.

The midline episiotomy, while being the easiest to repair and the most comfortable for the patient, does run the risk of extending to involve the anal sphincter and rectum in a third-degree tear. Its use should be reserved for the experienced practitioner.

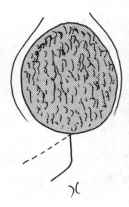

Fig. 6.12   Episiotomy sites.

> Whichever form of episiotomy is employed, it is important that the incision is made with the minimum of cuts and not multiple nibbles!

Once the episiotomy has been performed, delivery should follow. If there is undue bleeding from a vessel, it is a simple matter to apply an artery forceps. Otherwise pressure applied by a pad or even sponge-holding forceps should control bleeding.

Episiotomy repair (see Fig. 6.13)

This should follow delivery of the baby as soon as possible to prevent unnecessary blood loss.

(a) The patient is placed into the lithotomy position. If possible, do not attempt to repair an episiotomy simply with the patient lying on the delivery bed. It can become surprisingly awkward and take much longer to repair. A good light is essential. Scrub up. Swab the vulva downwards towards the perineum with chlorhexidine and apply the sterile drapes.

(b) Adequate analgesia is vital. The original perineal infiltration may have worn off. Be very gentle when determining the extent of the episiotomy. More local anaesthetic may be needed. Be sure to anaesthetize perineal skin, muscle, and finally vaginal skin edges.

(c) Gently place the tampon with the attached tape into the upper vagina above the apex of the vaginal incision.

(d) Place the first suture of 2–0 chromic catgut above the apex. This should not be too deep because of the proximity of the underlying rectal mucosa.

(e) The vaginal skin edges are now brought together with a continuous running stitch. The stitches should be less than 1 cm apart and without undue tension.

(f) When the vaginal skin edges are brought together at the introitus, bring the needle out under the skin so that the knot is underneath the skin edge. Tie off *gently*.

(g) Bring together the divided levator ani muscles with two or three interrupted sutures. Tie gently but firmly.

(h) Subcuticular suturing is preferable for the perineal skin although it is more complicated than interrupted suturing. Insert the needle under the perineal skin edge at the introitus, letting the needle tip emerge 0.5 cm below the skin edge. Clip the tail-end of the catgut with artery forceps.

(i) Use a continuous stitch (from side to side as a deep layer) until the lowest point of the incision on the perineum is reached. Here the stitch is brought out exactly under the skin edge.

(j) Reverse the direction of the needle. Insert stitch bites of less than 1 cm just under the skin edge, so that the beginning of each subcuticular stitch is exactly opposite the emerging end of the previous stitch on the other side. Be gentle and avoid undue tension to allow for possible oedema.

(k) The final subcuticular bite emerges at the introitus opposite the first stitch in step (h) above. Release the catgut from the artery forceps and gently tie the two ends together.

(l) Remove the tampon. Perform a vaginal examination to exclude a swab in the vagina (there should not have been any small swabs on the suture trolley in the first place).

(m) Perform a rectal examination to ensure that the suture at the apex of the vaginal incision has not penetrated the rectum. Clean the perineum. A soft sanitary pad should be applied and the legs gently and slowly lowered together to the horizontal position.

Sadly, some women say after the experience of their pregnancy and delivery, 'Never again!' That is bad enough, but if a woman reaches the same decision on account of the trauma and misery caused by a poorly carried-out and sutured episiotomy, it would be a damning indictment.

Perineal tears

Perineal tears may result from a poorly controlled delivery of the head as in precipitate labour. They are also associated with the delivery of large babies with large shoulders.

Classification of perineal tears

First degree tear: superficial tear of vaginal skin or fourchette.

Second degree tear: a deep tear involving perineal muscles and occasionally fibres of the anal sphincter; there may be other vaginal lacerations.

Third degree tear: an extension of either an episiotomy or second degree tear completely through the sphincter to involve rectal mucosa.

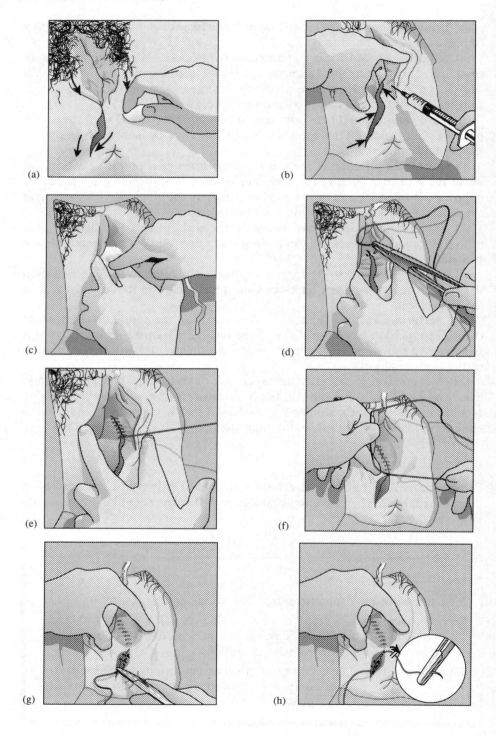

(a)

(b)

(c)

(d)

(e)

(f)

(g)

(h)

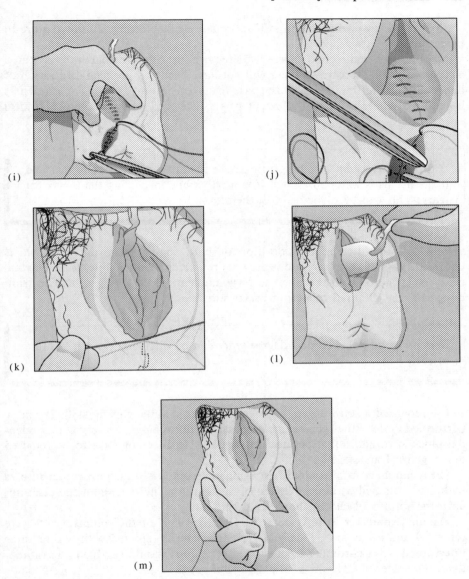

Fig. 6.13   Suturing an episiotomy.

First degree tears that are superficial and are not bleeding do not require to be sutured.

All other first and second degree tears require suturing. The patient is prepared as for episiotomy repair. As there will not have been any perineal infiltration of lignocaine before the tear as in the case of an episiotomy, particular gentleness is required in determining the extent of the tear and while instilling the local anaesthetic.

> If there is persistent bleeding from above the apex of the vaginal tear and if the uterus is well contracted, it is worth while inspecting the cervix for tears. This can be difficult. Seek help.

It is essential that good opposition of both vaginal skin and perineum is obtained. Vaginal skin lacerations are repaired along identical lines to the vaginal repair of episiotomy. If the edges of a vaginal tear are very ragged, a little 'trimming' may be required to permit easier suturing.

> Repairs of complex second degree tears can be difficult. Do not hesitate to seek help.

The repair of a third degree tear requires considerable clinical skill. It can be performed under either general anaesthesia, epidural block, or very good pudendal block with additional perineal infiltration. It does not *have* to be repaired under general anaesthetic.

The rectal mucosa is repaired first using interrupted 2–0 chromic catgut sutures with the knots tied within the lumen of the rectum. The spacing of these sutures 'mirrors' sutures placed in the vaginal skin.

The anal sphincter is now repaired. One torn half of the sphincter will have retracted and needs to be localized. The sphincter is repaired with two or three interrupted No. 1 chromic catgut sutures. The anus should be able to accommodate one finger at the end of the sphincter repair.

The third degree tear has now been converted into a second degree tear which is repaired in the normal way described above.

It is essential that the rectal mucosa is very carefully repaired. It must be repaired as a separate layer from the vaginal skin in order to avoid the complication of a recto-vaginal fistula.

A low fibre diet is necessary for the next week. Constipation must be avoided, but do not use any oil-based aperient. Lactulose 15 ml twice daily or Normacol 10 ml twice daily should be given.

If a woman has had a successful repair of a third degree tear, pressure on the

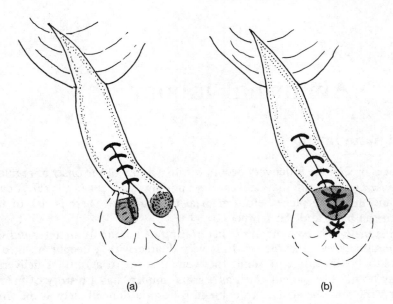

(a)

(b)

Fig. 6.14 Repair of third degree tear involving anal sphincter and rectum.

repair site must not be permitted, in any future vaginal delivery. It is essential
to carry out an elective episiotomy angled away from the original repair. Very
occasionally, the complication of a recto-vaginal fistula can follow a third degree
repair. Following a deferred successful repair of a fistula, it may be preferable
to consider elective Caesarean section for future deliveries.

If an episiotomy or repair (not third degree) breaks down during the puerperium, do not be tempted to rush in and carry out a secondary repair. It is far
better to carry out saline baths three times per day and defer surgery for 3
months. Superficial breakdown will heal by secondary intention if the perineum
is kept clean with saline baths.

7   Abnormal labour

Precipitate labour

Labour is precipitate if delivery occurs within 4 hours of the onset of regular contractions. The risks are that delivery does not always occur in the safest environment and may take place before medical help arrives. There is risk of trauma to both the baby and the mother.

Occasionally it is possible to predict precipitate labour. If an antenatal vaginal examination shows that the cervix is very dilated with a deeply engaged head, it is undoubtedly safest to admit the woman so as to avoid her delivering on the way home! If a patient, such as a grand multip, has a history of precipitate labours, she must be advised to come into hospital immediately at the first sign of labour. Admission at 38–39 weeks should be considered, particularly if she lives some distance away from the hospital, or during the winter when grim weather may make it difficult for her to reach the hospital in time.

When in labour, the woman must not be left unattended. Delivery can occur with surprising rapidity.

There is rarely a need to augment labour. Syntocinon may cause tetanic contractions and severe fetal hypoxia.

Prolonged labour

In normal labour, once the latent phase of cervical effacement is completed with the cervix usually being at least 3 cm dilated, it is possible to roughly predict how labour will progress. An 'action line' for either the primiparous or multiparous patient can be drawn onto the partogram, based from the first record of cervical dilatation. The rate of progress in labour is determined by the rate of descent of the presenting part of the fetus and the rate of dilatation of the cervix. During the active phase of labour, the rate of cervical dilatation for the primiparous patient is at least 1 cm per hour and for the multiparous 2 cm per hour. If there is any deviation from the predicted progress in labour, this will alert the observer so that appropriate action can be undertaken. In practice this means that labour may be considered to be abnormal if cervical dilatation lags more than 2 hours behind the expected rate of dilatation.

At least 90 per cent of primiparous and multiparous patients will reach full dilatation of the cervix within 10 hours and 6 hours respectively. If established labour continues for 18 hours or more it is prolonged.

Causes of prolonged labour

- abnormal uterine action
- occipito-posterior presentation
- cephalo-pelvic disproportion.

Abnormal uterine action

All forms of abnormal uterine action have one feature in common: contractions are inefficient and do not result in progressive dilatation of the cervix. The contractions may be weak and infrequent (hypotonic), irregular but strong (incoordinate), or frequent and strong (hypertonic).

It is essential to exclude cephalo-pelvic disproportion and malpresentations as a cause for the uterine inertia.

Hypotonic inertia is a common feature of labour when the uterus is overdistended as in cases of polyhydramnios and multiple pregnancy. The use of opiate analgesia too soon in labour can cause a reduction and slowing of uterine activity.

During **incoordinate uterine activity,** the cervix fails to dilate adequately in spite of the contractions being strong when they do occur.

Hypertonic uterine activity produces contractions which are so strong and frequent that they cause major distress to both mother and fetus.

Spontaneous hypertonic contractions must be considered to be due to placental abruption.

A more commonly seen major cause is the excessive use of oxytocic drugs in multiparous patients with unrecognized disproportion. Syntocinon infusion rates are sometimes inappropriately high. The risk of persistently strong contractions under these circumstances is uterine rupture.

BEWARE hypertonic contractions in multiparous patients. Disproportion due to malpresentation is the likely cause.

Management of abnormal uterine action

With the exception of hypertonic contractions, the management of the remaining forms of inefficient uterine activity are essentially the same. If there is no immediate concern over fetal well-being, **maternal distress** characterized by exhaustion, tachycardia, pyrexia, and significant ketonuria must be alleviated. The ketosis will be linked to the probable dehydration and starvation of the woman throughout a long labour. Both calories and fluid are required to correct this and are best provided by giving a rapid intravenous infusion of one litre 10 per cent dextrose. Thereafter a recurrence of ketosis is prevented with a dextrose infusion.

Cephalo-pelvic disproportion must be excluded. In multiparous patients this is most likely to be due to a malpresentation such as a brow presentation. Vaginal examination and erect lateral pelvimetry should reveal the true state of affairs.

If there is no contraindication to labour continuing, fetal well-being must be monitored with continuous CTG by scalp clip and an epidural or adequate opiate analgesia given to provide some rest for the woman. A syntocinon infusion is commenced. If labour still fails to progress satisfactorily, or if fetal distress should occur, delivery by Caesarean section will be required.

Remember that the pattern of contractions recorded by the external tocometer on a CTG tracing does not reflect the strength of those contractions.

If spontaneous hypertonic contractions occur there will usually be associated fetal distress. As the likely diagnosis will be abruptio placentae, the only opportunity of obtaining a live baby will be by emergency Caesarean section.

When hypertonic uterine activity is caused by abruptio placentae, NEVER give tocolytic drugs to reduce the frequency of contractions.

When hypertonic contractions are due to excessive syntocinon, the first immediate step is to stop the infusion while the situation is reassessed. A malpresentation is likely in multiparous patients and must be excluded.

Don't forget the possibility of a full bladder preventing progress in labour. An undiagnosed placenta praevia or pelvic fibroid will also prevent descent of the head.

If there is a past history of cervical surgery, cervical stenosis may result. On examination the cervix may at first thought to be fully dilated but is then found to be paper-thin and stretched over the fetal head with a pin-hole cervical os. The risk is of uterine rupture unless the cervix can be encouraged to dilate. Occasionally the thinned-out but stenosed and fibrotic external os can be dilated with persistent yet controlled digital pressure. If this fails, Caesarean section is the only alternative.

Occipito-posterior (OP) presentation

An OP presentation is the commonest cause of a high head at term in a primigravid patient. In this malposition of the vertex, the head is deflexed with the wider occipito-frontal diameter of 11.3 cm presenting instead of the well-flexed sub-occipito–bregmatic diameter of 9.5 cm.

On abdominal inspection, there is usually a flattened 'plateau' appearance to the anterior abdominal wall as the curvature of the fetal back is alongside the maternal spine. Fetal limbs are easily palpable whereas the fetal back cannot be felt with ease. On vaginal examination, the anterior fontanelle is anterior behind the symphysis pubis and the posterior fontanelle may only just be reached posteriorly.

The deflexed head is not a good presenting part, being ovoid in shape rather than the round shape brought about by good flexion. In common with other malpresentations, the membranes may rupture early as the first sign of labour.

As long as the contractions are adequate, the head will tend to enter the pelvic brim transversely. Descent, flexion, and rotation will occur, bringing the occiput into an anterior position. Delivery should occur normally.

If the contractions are inadequate, the head will tend to remain in an OP position. A larger diameter therefore presents and more time is required to bring about descent. As the head fits poorly against the lower segment and cervix, the stimulation to produce contractions remains sub-optimal. The head does not flex. Characteristic 'jam pot' moulding occurs and considerable caput may develop. In the absence of good contractions, the head will remain in a persistent OP position and be delivered face to pubes. A persistent OP presentation is also common in the patient with an android pelvis as the transverse diameters of the pelvis are narrower than the antero-posterior diameters. The occiput tends to remain posterior as there is more room posteriorly.

When there is flexion, the occiput will reach the gutter mechanism of the pelvic floor first and be rotated anteriorly. In those cases where the head engages transversely and contractions are inadequate, flexion will not occur. The deflexed head is unable to stimulate rotation as both the occiput and sinciput arrive on the pelvic floor together. The head will remain in a transverse position. Occasionally, deep transverse arrest of the head will occur.

Management of OP labour

Labour can only be contemplated if the pelvis is clinically adequate. Labour will tend to last several hours longer than a normal labour unless flexion can be brought about by means of adequate contractions.

Requirements for OP labour

- adequate analgesia
- adequate contractions
- adequate hydration.

Analgesia is best provided by means of an epidural block. OP labours often produce considerable low back pain owing to the pressure of the occiput against the rectum. Unless relieved, this can cause the woman to start involuntary pushing late in the first stage of labour.

A syntocinon infusion will provide adequate stimulation. Intravenous fluids will prevent dehydration and ketosis. Continuous fetal heart monitoring by CTG is essential.

If labour does not progress satisfactorily in spite of adequate stimulation, Caesarean section is indicated.

As long as labour progresses satisfactorily, the second stage will be reached without undue delay. The head will either undergo long rotation on the pelvic floor to bring the occiput anterior, or will remain as a persistent OP and be delivered face to pubes.

Delay in the second stage of labour is a common feature of these labours. With an epidural it is sensible to wait until the head has reached the perineum before maternal effort commences.

Even though caput and moulding presents at the vulva, do not be fooled into thinking that the head is on the pelvic floor. This is particularly important when considering operative delivery.

If maternal effort is inadequate to deliver the baby or, as is often the case, she is simply too tired, operative delivery will be required.

Options for operative delivery of OP presentation

- forceps (direct OP)
- rotation with Kjellands forceps
- manual rotation/forceps
- ventouse
- Caesarean section.

The majority of OP presentations and transverse arrests are able to be delivered via the vaginal route. Always use a large J-shaped episiotomy to avoid extension into the rectum. If any difficulty is invisaged, carry out the forceps in theatre as a 'trial of forceps'.

Caesarean section is a safer option than a difficult delivery.

Cephalo-pelvic disproportion

One of the major aims of antenatal care is the detection of cephalo-pelvic disproportion (p. 26 and p. 100). Every primigravida should have had a clinical assessment of the pelvis by the 38th week. In the case of multiparous women, it is easy to be lulled into a false sense of security by an earlier successful vaginal delivery. However, there is a tendency for each successive baby to be larger. When labour is prolonged, cephalo-pelvic disproportion must be considered as a possible cause.

When labour is prolonged, exclude cephalo-pelvic disproportion and malpresentations before stimulating labour with oxytocics.

A vaginal examination by an experienced clinician will usually allow diagnosis of a malpresentation and permit clinical assessment of the pelvis. This should be backed up by erect lateral pelvimetry. Cephalo-pelvic disproportion in the absence of a malpresentation will result in delivery by Caesarean section. Any malpresentation is managed by normal clinical practice.

Trial of labour

The term 'trial of labour' is frequently misused to describe a 'trial of vaginal delivery' in a breech labour or a 'trial of scar'. A trial of labour applies *only* to the highly controlled, supervised attempt at vaginal delivery in the presence of borderline cephalo-pelvic disproportion at the pelvic brim. If the pelvic brim can be successfully negotiated by the fetal head, there should be no further bar to delivery. There is never a place for a double trial such as a trial of scar *and* a trial of labour.

Pre-conditions for trial of labour

(1) the presentation must be cephalic;

(2) no malpresentation or malposition of the head;

(3) no uterine scars;

(4) no pelvic outlet contracture;

(5) no additional maternal factor:
　　PIH
　　diabetes
　　cardiac disease
　　elderly primigravida
　　poor obstetric history;

(6) no concern over fetal well-being:
　　IUGR
　　rhesus iso-immunization.

Once a woman has been selected for a trial of labour, there are strict guidelines regarding the conduct of the trial.

Conduct of trial of labour

(1) ideally the onset of labour should be spontaneous;

(2) amniotomy is performed;

(3) continuous fetal heart monitoring is carried out;

(4) adequate intravenous hydration;

(5) augmentation with syntocinon is performed if indicated;

(6) an epidural is given;

(7) blood is cross-matched.

There is little point in putting an absolute time limit on a trial of labour. As long as labour progresses satisfactorily with descent of the head and dilatation of the cervix, and there are no concerns for fetal or maternal well-being, the trial may continue. The trial of labour is only completed at full dilatation with the head engaged in the pelvis. The second stage is conducted normally. Many trials of labour are not completed but are interrupted owing to fetal distress or a failure to progress adequately in labour. Caesarean section is then the only alternative.

Trial of forceps

This term refers to the conduct of a forceps delivery when there is doubt about the adequacy of the pelvic outlet. When the baby is large or a pelvic assessment inaicates a narrow sub-pubic angle, the need for forceps delivery for delay in the second stage can be predicted. In such cases, it is safer to carry out the forceps delivery in theatre with the intention of proceeding to Caesarean section if problems should arise. An episiotomy should only be performed if the prospects for a successful vaginal delivery are good.

Management of breech presentation in labour

The antenatal management of breech presentation and the antenatal selection of patients potentially suitable for a vaginal breech delivery has been discussed (p. 105). It must always be made clear to the woman that circumstances may alter at any time and indicate a change of course and Caesarean section. For example, if induction of labour is indicated and the breech is very high and/or the cervix very unfavourable, it may well be considered preferable to deliver abdominally than to attempt cervical 'ripening' and hope for descent of the breech.

> Any concern over the outcome of a breech labour is an indication to reassess the original intention of achieving a vaginal delivery.

Induction of labour in a breech presentation is no different from induction for cephalic presentations. When the breech is flexed there is a greater chance of cord prolapse at amniotomy because the presenting part does not fit as snugly in the pelvis as the extended breech. An epidural block is an ideal form of analgesia during a breech labour, especially during the second stage when forceps are commonly used to deliver the 'after-coming' head. If a non-emergency Caesarean section is indicated during labour, the established epidural may avoid the need for a general anaesthetic.

> If a breech labour is significantly preterm, vaginal delivery may well be contraindicated. Labour should ONLY be contemplated if an epidural is given.

An epidural will reduce the often overwhelming urge, especially in a multiparous woman, to push late in the first stage — which can result in the baby being delivered up to the neck through an incompletely dilated cervix.

Fetal heart monitoring is carried out either by using an external ultrasound transducer or by applying a scalp clip to the fetal buttock. Fetal blood sampling from the buttock does not present a problem, although the blood flow is reduced in comparison to the scalp.

> If there is concern about fetal well-being during any stage of a breech labour, deliver by Caesarean section.

It should never be assumed that the passage of meconium in a breech labour is simply due to pressure on the fetal abdomen.

> An anoxic fetus may pass meconium regardless of its presentation.

The assessment of progress in a breech labour is the same as for a cephalic presentation, namely the dilatation of the cervix and descent of the breech. The duration of labour is also the same. Indeed, prolonged labour in a breech presentation is an indication to proceed to abdominal delivery rather than to augment labour with syntocinon. Augmented breech labours are associated with a higher perinatal mortality rate.

The diagnosis of the second stage of labour cannot be made easily by vaginal examination. The fact that no cervix can be felt does not exclude the possibility of there being a rim of cervix through which the breech has passed. The fetal scrotum may present at the introitus for some time before full dilatation is reached.

> The second stage is only diagnosed when the anterior buttock is visible.

DO NOT encourage the patient to push until the second stage has been diagnosed. This is especially important in the multiparous patient or the patient with a very preterm labour. It can be suprisingly easy for a multiparous patient to push the relatively narrow breech through an 8 cm dilated cervix.

Once the second stage has been reached, preparations should be made for an assisted breech delivery. It is essential that this is conducted by an experienced obstetrician. A paediatrician should be available and the anaesthetist standing by.

The patient is placed in lithotomy. The perineum is cleaned and draped. The bladder is catheterized. If an epidural has not been used, a pudendal block is inserted (as described on p. 164).

Maternal effort is now encouraged. When the anterior buttock reaches and distends the perineum, an episiotomy is carried out. The episiotomy is performed at this early stage to straighten the vagina and so assist in the delivery of the breech which is unable to flex as well as the head on the neck. There are also no vital structures such as the umbilical cord or fetal neck to get in the way, which may occur if the episiotomy is delayed until required for the delivery of the 'after-coming' head.

With maternal effort the breech is now delivered. In the flexed breech, the feet will present beneath the breech and the legs will be delivered spontaneously. In the extended breech each thigh is gently abducted and the knee flexed so that the foot is drawn down through the maternal pelvis to the perineum and delivered. As the abdomen is delivered, a loop of cord is gently drawn down so as to take tension off the umbilicus.

> After the fetal abdomen has been delivered, the breech delivery must be completed within 10 minutes.

The abdomen and legs should be wrapped in a sterile towel to allow the baby to be held with more safety. The baby is supported by holding the pelvis and not the abdomen so as to avoid injury to fetal organs such as the liver and spleen.

> No traction is *ever* applied to the fetal abdomen.

The only action of the operator at this point is to ensure that the fetal back remains anterior and to support the weight of the baby. As the delivery progresses, the arms should be looked for beneath the chest and be delivered spontaneously. If the arms cannot be seen, they will be extended above the baby's head, probably as a result of traction during an earlier stage of the delivery. The arms can invariably be delivered with ease using Løvset's manoeuvre (Fig. 7.1).

The principle behind this beautiful technique is that if the baby is rotated through 180 degrees while applying downward traction on the pelvis, one of the baby's shoulders will then be lying within the hollow of the sacrum. On rotating the baby back again, that (posterior) shoulder will present beneath the symphysis pubis. The arm can then be delivered. The opposite shoulder will now be lying within the pelvis, and a repeat rotation will allow it to be delivered beneath the symphysis. The arms are now included in the sterile towel so that they will not be in the way during the delivery of the head.

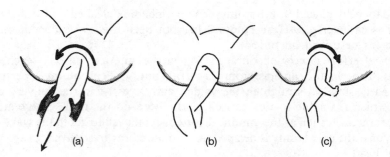

Fig. 7.1 Lovset's manoeuvre; (a) downward traction on the baby's pelvis and rotation through 180°; (b) the shoulder that had been posterior now presents beneath the symphysis pubis; (c) after delivery of the arm, the procedure is reversed so as to bring the other shoulder beneath the symphsis.

When the hair on the nape of the baby's neck is visible, an assistant should now support and elevate the baby approximately 45 degrees above the horizontal so that forceps can be applied directly to the 'after-coming' head from beneath the baby's body. Minimal traction should be applied so that the head is virtually eased out of the pelvis. As soon as the mouth is visible it should be possible to aspirate the pharynx.

There are two non-instrumental methods of delivering the baby's head but these do not give as safe or as good a control as forceps. In the Burns–Marshall technique, the operator elevates the baby in an arc while also applying outward traction. At 45 degrees above the horizontal the baby's mouth should become visible. While continuing to provide traction, the perineum is guarded to prevent too sudden a delivery of the head. In the Mauriceau–Smellie–Veit manoeuvre of shoulder–jaw traction, the baby is laid along the length of the operator's forearm. The operator's index and middle fingers are placed on the baby's cheek-bones and drawn downwards to increase flexion. Traction from within the the baby's mouth with the index finger is not so effective and can traumatize the mandible. The other hand is placed on the baby's shoulders and gentle pressure is applied to the occiput to also encourage flexion. Once the occiput is delivered elevation of the baby's body will allow delivery of the head.

A breech extraction using groin and pelvic traction is rarely indicated, unless a speedy delivery suddenly becomes necessary while the second stage is under way. It should only be performed by a very experienced operator. The baby's arms will invariably become extended above the head and Løvset's manoeuvre will be necessary. In these circumstances, delivery of the head must still be controlled and gentle. In breech deliveries there is no time for the head to adapt to the shape of the mother's pelvis by moulding, as the head is still above the pelvic brim while the arms are being delivered. Delivery of the head is therefore always accomplished by initial compression followed by carefully controlled decompression.

If delivery of the head is sudden or uncontrolled, tentorial tears and fatal intracerebral haemorrhage may result.

Breech delivery by Caesarean section is always by breech extraction and generally involves the same principles already described. The use of Wrigley's forceps permits very controlled delivery of the baby's head through the uterine incision.

There are two major nightmares that can arise during a breech delivery.

The first is the baby that has been delivered up to the neck through an **incompletely dilated cervix**. This is usually associates with preterm labours, especially of very multiparous woman, without epidural block who have been unable to resist the urge to push before full dilatationis achieved. It is sometimes possible to apply forceps within the cervical rim and, if the baby is small, as is usually the case, delivery is possible. A combination of the Mauriceau–Smellie–Veit technique combined with supra-pubic pressure may also be tried. If these manoeuvres should fail, the only other option is to incise the cervix. The incisions are made with scissors at the two, six, and ten o'clock positions on the cervix (avoiding three and nine o'clock sites as these can extend upwards to involve the uterine arteries). The risks of such incisions are that any of them may extend upwards and be very haemorrhagic and difficult to repair.

The second major complication is the realization that there is **cephalo-pelvic disproportion** because the head cannot be delivered. The Mauriceau–Smellie–Veit manoeuvre combined with supra-pubic pressure may be successful but, if not, the only realistic option for obtaining a live baby is symphysiotomy. Caesarean section has been performed in this grim situation, but under these circumstances it is extremely difficult as the baby has to be reintroduced into the uterus from the vagina.

Hydrocephalus leading to disproportion should not have escaped antenatal detection. However, if this diagnosis does become apparent in labour, cerebral decompression of the baby either through the skull or via an associated spina bifida will permit vaginal delivery.

Management of twin pregnancy in labour

The risks of preterm labour occuring in multiple pregnancy have already been commented upon (pp. 107–10). If labour becomes established before 32 weeks, delivery should be by Caesarean section.

If labour does not occur spontaneously, induction is generally carried out at 38 weeks. It is, of course, essential that the first twin has a longitudinal lie. The method of induction will depend upon the 'favourability' of the cervix.

The over-distended uterus of a multiple pregnancy, is, as a rule, an inefficient contractor in labour. Left to its own devices, labour will tend to be prolonged.

The delayed first stage leads to a delayed second stage and, most dangerous of all, a delayed third stage with the attendant risks of postpartum haemorrhage.

> A syntocinon infusion is strongly recommended for all twin labours.

Both twins should be monitored simultaneously, the first twin by means of a fetal electrode and the second twin by an external ultrasound transducer. Modern cardiotocography machines permit both fetal hearts to be recorded on the same monitor. There is, therefore, the opportunity for detecting fetal distress in the second twin and taking appropriate emergency action.

Instrumental deliveries are commonly required, especially if one of the twins presents as a breech. Although a pudendal block will give adequate analgesia for forceps deliveries, an epidural block given in established labour is ideal as it provides excellent pain relief, especially in the second stage when operative delivery may be required.

Delivery of the first twin should be as for any singleton pregnancy. The cord clamps used for each twin should be tagged in some way so that retrospectively each baby and its cord and placenta can be identified.

> Apart from the syntocinon infusion, NO OXYTOCIC is given until *after the second twin has been delivered.*

After the first twin has been delivered, the lie of the second twin is determined immediately and the fetal heart is checked. The commonest presentations of twins are:

cephalic/cephalic
cephalic/breech
breech/cephalic
breech/breech
cephalic/transverse
breech/transverse
transverse/cephalic, breech, transverse

(Obviously, if the lie of the first twin is transverse, the only safe method of delivery is by elective Caesarean section.)

If the lie of the second twin is other than longitudinal, external cephalic version is carried out. With the next contraction, maternal effort is strongly encouraged so that the presenting part descends into the pelvis. Amniotomy is usually carried out during this contraction. Delivery should then follow normally as for a singleton cephalic or breech presentation.

Delivery of the second twin is not always straightforward. Very occasionally it is not possible to carry out an external version and the lie remains persistently oblique or transverse. Other complications include the head that remains high, cord prolapse, and fetal distress. In such circumstances the *experienced obstetrician* may carry out an internal podalic version. There is so much room in the uterus after the delivery of the first twin that this manoeuvre should be accomplished without undue difficulty. First the heel and then the foot of the baby is sought and brought down into the pelvis. A breech extraction (p. 196) is then performed. The only alternative to internal version and breech extraction is Caesarean section for the second twin.

The combination of a lax uterus that tends to contract poorly and a double-sized placental surface area is a good recipe for postpartum haemorrhage. To reduce the chances of this complication occurring, intravenous ergometrine 0.25 mg should be given immediately after the delivery of the second twin. *When the uterus is well contracted*, the placentae are delivered by controlled cord traction. The intravenous injection of ergometrine is repeated. A high dosage syntocinon infusion (40 units in 500 ml 5 per cent dextrose) is given over the next 4 hours to maintain good uterine contraction.

Undiagnosed twins will be a rare event in modern obstetric practice. Beware the large, difficult-to-examine, unbooked patient who turns up in labour having had no antenatal care! The risk, of course, is that syntometrine or ergometrine is given 'routinely' with the delivery of the anterior shoulder of the baby. Only difficulty in the third stage with a placenta that refuses to be delivered, a very large uterus and subsequent vaginal examination reveals that there is a second occupant! Amniotomy and immediate vaginal delivery should be attempted. An emergency Caesarean section may be required if the uterus remains firmly contracted and fetal distress of the second twin develops.

The rarest problem that can occur in a twin delivery is that of 'locked twins'. This can occur when the presentation is breech/cephalic and the head of the breech becomes trapped above the head of the second baby. Under epidural block or general anaesthesia it should be possible to manipulate the head of the second twin and displace it above the head of the breech. Obviously, time is of the essence in this situation.

Management of face presentation

When the fetal head is fully extended on the neck the face will present. It is unusual to diagnose a face presentation antenatally, unless found incidentally at vaginal examination for pelvic assessment. Face presentation most commonly presents on the labour ward and complicates less than 1 per cent of labours. On vaginal examination the examiner may be disconcerted to find an irregular presenting part formed by the eyes, nose, and mouth. While it is possible to confuse the mouth with the anus, the clue to making the diagnosis is to recognize the fetal nose.

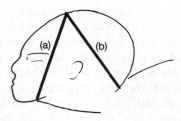

Fig. 7.2   Face presentation; (a) submento-bregmatic diameter (9.5 cm); (b) subocci-pito-bregmatic diameter (9.5 cm).

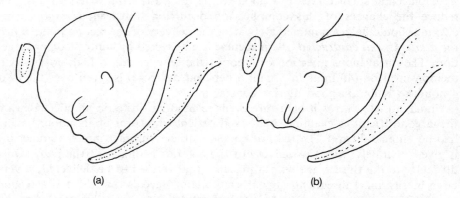

Fig. 7.3   Face presentation; (a) mento-posterior; (b) mento-anterior.

> The nose is the only part of the fetal anatomy which has two little holes side by side!

If there is uncertainty about the presentation, a pelvic CT scan or erect lateral pelvimetry will be of value.

> When an unbooked patient who has had no antenatal care is admitted in labour with a face presentation, remember that the anencephalic head will always present as a face. An erect lateral pelvic X-ray will establish the diagnosis.

Another rare cause of face presentation is an anterior neck tumour which extends the fetal head.

A face presentation is generally a very good presenting part, as the sub-mento–bregmatic diameter of 9.5 cm is the same as the sub-occipito–bregmatic diameter when there is full flexion (Fig. 7.2).

When the chin is anterior (mento-anterior) the head will be delivered by flexion on the neck. However, if the chin is posterior (mento-posterior), the baby will be undeliverable without assistance as the hyperextended head cannot extend any further to permit the face to 'climb the perineum' during the second stage of labour (Fig. 7.3).

Unless the mento-posterior position can be rotated to the mento-anterior by Kjelland's forceps, the only alternative is Caesarean section. This is the only safe option if there are any other factors leading to concern for fetal well-being.

If vaginal delivery is contemplated, this should only be undertaken by an experienced obstetrician.

After delivery, the baby's face will appear very bruised and oedematous as the face is unable to undergo moulding in labour. The hyperextension will persist for a few days but the muscle tone in the neck will gradually diminish. The mother must be warned of the dramatic degree of facial bruising before delivery and be reassured.

Management of brow presentation

A brow presentation may be diagnosed antenatally when investigating a high head at term. A pelvic CT scan or erect lateral pelvimetry will confirm the diagnosis. On vaginal examination, the head may be high with a poorly applied cervix and the anterior fontanelle, supra-orbital ridges and eyes will be felt. Unless the baby is small or the pelvis is cavernous, the *persistent* brow presentation is unlikely to engage, as the presenting vertico–mental diameter of 13.5 cm is greater than any of the normal diameters of the pelvis (Fig. 7.4).

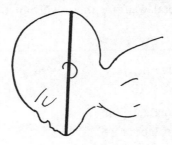

Fig. 7.4 Brow presentation. Vertico-mental diameter 13.5 cm.

However, the antenatal diagnosis of a brow may only be a temporary finding as the head may extend further and become a face presentation or flex into an occipito-posterior presentation. The incidence of brow presentation in labour is approximately 1 in 1500 deliveries.

> If there is any concern over fetal well-being, the persistent brow presentation should be delivered by Caesarean section.

If there are no contraindications, a *short* trial of labour (see p. 191) may be considered reasonable by an experienced obstetrician. The presence of contractions can change the presentation by bringing about flexion or extension. As long as there is progress in a closely supervised and continuously monitored labour, with good descent of the head and cervical dilatation, labour can be permitted to continue.

> If the brow presentation persists or progress in labour is poor, delivery by Caesarean section is indicated to avoid obstructed labour and uterine rupture.

Compound presentation

Occasionally on vaginal examination in labour, the fetal hand may be felt alongside the head. In the majority of such cases the hand can be pushed up past the head during a contraction and the problem is resolved.

Operative delivery

Some patients will be booked to have an elective operative delivery. For the remainder, if labour is progressing normally and there is no immediate concern for either maternal or fetal welfare, there will not be any need for operative intervention.

> Indications for operative delivery
>
> - fetal distress
> - maternal distress or exhaustion
> - failure to progress in labour
> - elective procedure for maternal or fetal conditions.

Operative deliveries include the use of forceps, ventouse (vacuum extractor), Caesarean section, and (rarely in the UK) symphysiotomy.

> It cannot be over-stressed that expertise with instrumental deliveries can only be gained by personal experience combined with good teaching and supervision.

Forceps deliveries

Forceps are chiefly used to assist and often expedite the delivery of the baby during the second stage of labour. Forceps are of two main types. They are designed to apply either direct traction to deliver the fetal head or initial rotation of a malpositioned head prior to traction and delivery.

> Indications for forceps delivery
>
> - fetal distress in second stage of labour
> - delay in the second stage of labour
> - as an elective procedure to avoid maternal effort:
>   dural tap at epidural
>   severe hypertensive disease
>   respiratory disease
>   following a successful 'trial of scar' once second stage of labour
>   is reached
>   cardiac patients
> - as an elective procedure to protect the fetal skull and brain from compression and decompression forces at delivery:
>   after-coming head at breech delivery
>   preterm delivery before 36 weeks
> - occasionally to assist delivery of the head through the uterine incision at Caesarean section.

There are two main types of traction forceps. The long curved forceps (such as Neville Barnes, Simpson's, Milne Murray) are used when the head is in the mid-cavity of the pelvis. The short curved forceps (such as Wrigley's forceps) can only be used when the head is on the perineum and simply requires a 'lift out', or to assist the delivery of the head at Caesarean section. Both the long and the short curved forceps have a cephalic curve to accommodate the fetal head and a pelvic curve which follows the curve of the sacrum during traction and delivery.

Rotation forceps (Kjelland's forceps), while having a cephalic curve to accommodate the head, have very little pelvic curve. This means that rotation of an occipito-posterior or occipito-transverse position to occipito-anterior is possible without inflicting trauma to the vaginal walls. There is an unfortunate tendency to regard Kjelland's forceps as 'dangerous'—but so is a scalpel in inexperienced hands. There is no doubt that the skilled use of Kjelland's forceps exemplifies the true 'art' of obstetrics.

Conditions to be fulfilled before the application of forceps

Absolute conditions
(1) The cervix **must** be fully dilated;
(2) the head **must** be engaged (at or below the level of the ischial spines). BEWARE A LARGE CAPUT AT OR BELOW THE SPINES masking what is really a high head;
(3) the position of the head **must** be known;
(4) the membranes **must** be ruptured.

Additional conditions in good obstetric practice
(1) Adequate anaesthesia **must** be given;
(2) the uterus **must** be contracting;
(3) the bladder **must** be empty.

Many women have a dread of forceps and fear that their use can only lead to damage of their baby's head at delivery. One of the roles of antenatal care is to dispel such fears. It is useful to explain that forceps do in fact fulfil a protective function and have a 'crash helmet' effect.

The woman must be told clearly and simply of the need for intervention with forceps and be given a brief explanation of what to expect. REASSURANCE IS ESSENTIAL.

Forceps deliveries are carried out with the patient in the lithotomy position. Using full aseptic techniques, the perineum is cleaned and draped. The bladder is emptied. A vaginal examination is performed to confirm that the cervix is fully dilated and to determine the station of the head in relation to the ischial spines and the position of the head. It is unusual to reach the second stage of labour with intact membranes, but if this is the case, amniotomy is performed.

While all of the absolute conditions listed above are essential, it is obvious that forceps cannot be applied with safety unless the position of the head is accurately

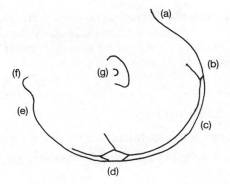

Fig. 7.5 Identifying landmarks on the fetal head at vaginal examination. (a) nape of neck; (b) hard occipital bone often overridden by parietal bones at posterior fontanelle; (c) 'ping-pong' effect of parietal bones along sagittal suture; (d) 'suture counting' at anterior fontanelle; (e) supra-orbital ridge and root of the nose; (f) nostril; (g) external auditory meatus.

known. It is usually easy to identify the long, straight, sagittal suture between the parietal bones unless there is a considerable degree of caput formation. The Y-shape formed by the lambdoid sutures running into the sagittal suture at the posterior fontanelle is difficult to miss when the head is well flexed. The occipital bone between the lambdoid sutures feels very much harder than the parietal bones which tend to overlap it. While it seems obvious that the anterior fontanelle is a diamond shape with four sutures running into it, it can be surprisingly difficult to identify. Outlining the shape of the fontanelle with two fingers and 'suture counting' around the diamond usually clarifies the situation. Feeling for the ear can be very helpful when caput seems to obliterate all other recognizable features. When the external auditory meatus has been identified and the true direction of the pinna of the ear determined (as it can be folded back on itself), the position of the head should be known (Fig. 7.5).

| If in doubt, NEVER GUESS. Seek help. |

A forceps delivery should be a relatively painless experience for the patient to undergo. There is *always* time to administer perineal infiltration and a pudendal block, even in the most dire case of fetal distress. This can probably be achieved with greater speed than a general anaesthetic. An epidural block that is already providing analgesia is ideal.

With the exceptions of a deeply engaged, direct occipito-posterior presentation where the head can be delivered 'face to pubes', and a mento-anterior face presentation, all other forceps deliveries must be performed with the occiput anterior. If the occiput is not anterior, the head must first be rotated into that position either with Kjelland's forceps or by manual rotation before any traction with forceps is applied.

Stages in traction forceps delivery

(1) assemble forceps and coat blades with obstetric cream;

(2) the right hand is inserted into the vagina between the baby's head and the left vaginal wall;

(3) the *left* handle of the assembled forceps is taken in the *left* hand;

(4) the handle is held parallel to the patient's right inguinal ligament and the tip of the blade is inserted into the *left* side of the vagina between the right hand and the baby's head;

(5) finger-tip pressure is then all that is required to insert the blade alongside the baby's head by gently bringing the handle down in an arc to the mid-line;

(6) the identical procedure is now carried out with the *right* blade; the *right* handle is taken in the *right* hand and the blade inserted into the *right* side of the vagina alongside the baby's head;

(7) the two forceps blades should now lock together *easily*;

Force must not be used to lock the blades

(8) the vaginal examination is repeated to ensure that the sagittal suture is still in the mid-line and that the occiput is anterior;

(9) combined with maternal effort during a contraction, gentle forearm traction is applied in a downwards direction; in the case of fetal distress do not await the next contraction but proceed with the delivery;

(10) as the head descends, the direction of traction becomes more horizontal;

(11) when the head reaches the perineum, an episiotomy is carried out; the direction of traction is now upwards;

(12) with delivery of the head, the forceps blades are unlocked and removed and the delivery continues normally.

See Fig. 7.6.

There is no place for the use of force in a forceps delivery, as the end result is likely to be a handicapped baby if it survives the obstetric insult. In the presence of severe fetal distress, especially if the episiotomy has been carried out too early,

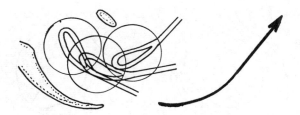

Fig. 7.6 Direction of traction during delivery with forceps. Note that when using Kjelland's forceps the handles do not rise above the horizontal plane.

the temptation to apply a 70 kg pull in order to achieve delivery must be resisted. Under such circumstances, the most difficult aspect of any forceps delivery is to remove the forceps and proceed to emergency Caesarean section and episiotomy repair. The nightmare of a further long delay can be avoided by recognizing those cases where there may be difficulty in carrying out a vaginal delivery. Panic can be avoided if the forceps attempt is carried out as a 'trial of forceps' in theatre with all preparations to hand to proceed to Caesarean section should the trial fail.

If there were difficulties in determining the position of the head before the application of forceps, it is always a useful exercise to feel the baby's head after delivery and with closed eyes identify the sutures and fontanelles.

Kjelland's rotation and delivery

An occipito-posterior or occipito-transverse position may lead to a longer second stage of labour while rotation of the head takes place in response to the combined effects of contractions and maternal effort. Intervention is often required to relieve maternal exhaustion and bring a delayed second stage to a satisfactory conclusion.

Kjelland's forceps are designed to be applied to the baby's head while it is still malpositioned so that after rotation to the occipito-anterior position, traction and delivery can be carried out without removing the forceps or needing to replace them with long curved forceps.

In normal labour, the head enters the pelvic brim in a transverse position by lateral inclination of the head on the neck so that the anterior parietal bone presents. This anterior asynclitism is a necessary requirement for the head to be able to negotiate the pelvic brim and pass the potential obstructions of the sacral promontory and symphysis pubis. Should the posterior parietal bone present (posterior asynclitism) then engagement and vaginal delivery may prove to be impossible. Caesarean section is the only alternative (Fig. 7.7).

The blades of Kjelland's forceps have a sliding lock which will correct asynclitism when present.

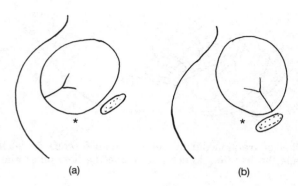

(a)   (b)

Fig. 7.7 (a) anterior asynclitism (anterior parietal bone presents*); (b) posterior asynclitism (posterior parietal bone presents*).

As in all forceps deliveries, adequate analgesia is essential. Many obstetricians feel that a Kjelland's rotation and delivery should only be performed under general anaesthetic or epidural block. However, a Kjelland's rotation can be beautifully performed with a good pudendal block, an indication of how little force is necessary to correct what may otherwise present a major problem.

Manual rotation versus Kjelland's forceps

Some obstetricians will favour manual rotation in preference to a Kjelland's forceps rotation, on the grounds that it is a safer procedure. However, manual rotation is not always an easy manoeuvre to accomplish, especially if the head is deep in the pelvis. It can be difficult to get a satisfactory grip on the head and it is necessary to over-rotate to prevent a recurrence of the malposition before applying long curved forceps to deliver the head. There is, also, usually some upwards displacement of the head.

In contrast, Kjelland's rotation can be carried out with greater ease and at a lower position in the pelvis than can be achieved at manual rotation. There is little chance of the malposition recurring while the forceps are still applied and there is minimal upward displacement of the head.

It is true that misapplied Kjelland's, excessive force during rotation, and an incorrect angle of traction can traumatize the baby and cause considerable damage to maternal soft tissues in the pelvis. But nobody would advocate such a misuse of the instrument. The use of Kjelland's forceps should be taught enthusiastically by experts in their use. It would be tragic if the skill of forceps rotation was lost in the mistaken belief that it was too dangerous to have a significant role to play in modern obstetrics.

Stages in Kjelland's forceps delivery

(1) assemble forceps and coat blades with obstetric cream;

(2) while it is possible to apply both blades directly, it is often easier to 'wander' the anterior blade over the baby's face and apply the posterior blade directly;

(3) to identify the anterior blade, hold the assembled forceps in the position they would occupy if they were already applied to the head in its current unrotated position; the directional knobs on each handle should point towards the occiput; the upper blade is the anterior blade;

(4) while memorizing the position that this blade will eventually occupy, it is gently inserted laterally alongside the the baby's face, guided by the second and third fingers of the other hand which have already been inserted into the vagina; these two fingers gently sweep the blade through a quarter of a circle over the baby's face to its intended position, while the handle of the blade is depressed;

(5) the posterior blade is applied directly to the head;

(6) the two blades should engage with ease and without any force (if the head is in the right occipito-lateral position, the handles will require to be crossed over each other, which is simple to do);

(7) if asynclitism is present, one blade will appear to be further in the vagina than the other; the sliding lock will correct the asynclitism;

(8) check the position of the head to ensure that the blades are correctly applied;

Keep the handles depressed during rotation and traction

(9) rotation of the head is carried out between contractions using no more than finger-tip pressure; sometimes slight traction is required before rotation can be achieved;

(10) check that the head is now occipito-anterior;

(11) an episiotomy is now performed;

(12) KEEPING THE HANDLES DOWN TOWARDS THE FLOOR (which is best achieved by kneeling), traction is gently applied until the occiput is seen beneath the symphysis; the handles are only now brought to the horizontal as traction continues;

(13) the head is delivered and the delivery completed.

Ventouse (vacuum extractor) delivery

The ventouse combines traction, using a specially-designed suction cup which fits onto the baby's scalp, with maternal effort to achieve delivery of the head. If rotation is required this will occur 'naturally' during the process of delivery. Some obstetricians will prefer to use the ventouse instead of forceps to carry out virtually all vaginal instrumental deliveries. However, the ventouse should not be seen as an alternative to the use of forceps, but as a complementary option.

The combination of symphysiotomy and ventouse has been well documented for remote areas of the world where access to Caesarean section may be difficult. Indeed, in such circumstances, it is far safer to *avoid* Caesarean section for cephalo-pelvic disproportion, because if a repeat Caesarean is not readily available in the next pregnancy, uterine scar rupture from obstructed labour may have lethal results.

The chief indication for using the ventouse is for delay in the second stage of labour. If there is fetal distress during the second stage, then a forceps delivery will generally be speedier. Unlike forceps, the ventouse can be applied before the cervix is fully dilated.

If the indication to deliver *before* full dilatation is prolonged labour, beware cephalo-pelvic disproportion.

Contraindications to using the ventouse

- cervix less than 7 cm dilated
- a high head (with the exception of the second twin)
- any suggestion of cephalo-pelvic disproportion
- fetal distress, as the ventouse generally takes longer than forceps
- face presentation, as the cup will cause trauma to the face
- preterm delivery before 34 weeks due to greater risk of cephalo-haematoma and intracranial bleeding.

There can be no doubt that in less experienced hands the ventouse is safer than forceps. Considerably less traction is required to achieve delivery. The operator does not need to do anything apart from apply traction correctly to rotate the baby's bead. One advantage of the ventouse is that the suction cup will come off the baby's head if excessive force is used. Therefore, there should be less likelihood of damage to maternal tissues.

A pudendal block should provide adequate analgesia for all cases. Perineal infiltration may be all the analgesia that is required if the head is on the perineum.

Stages in ventouse delivery

(1) Choose the largest cup which will fit with ease onto the baby's head; lubricate with an aqueous antiseptic rather than obstetric cream to reduce the chances of the cup slipping off the scalp;

(2) insert the cup into the vagina 'edgeways' and place it as far back as possible on the baby's head keeping to the mid-line; position the direction knob on the cup towards the occiput so that rotation can be appreciated;

(3) ensure that no cervix or vagina is included between the cup and fetal scalp;

(4) establish initial suction to $0.2 \, \text{kg/cm}^2$ and re-examine;

(5) continue to increase the suction by $0.1 \, \text{kg/cm}^2$ each minute to reach a suction pressure of $0.8 \, \text{kg/cm}^2$; if an electric pump is used it is possible to achieve the final suction pressure with greater speed; re-examine;

(6) traction is usually carried out with the right hand, placing the first and second fingers of the left hand on the cup and scalp respectively; the index finger ensures that the direction of traction is correct and that there is no sign of the cup becoming detached; the second finger assesses descent during traction;

(7) the direction of traction must remain perpendicular to the cup and not oblique, to avoid detachment;

(8) traction is carried out during contractions; in the second stage of labour, maternal effort is strongly encouraged; if contractions are infrequent, traction itself usually stimulates a contraction to begin; between the episodes of synchronized contractions, traction, and maternal effort, the head is held by the traction handle at the station it has reached so as not to lose the descent already gained;

(9) as in a forceps delivery, the direction of pull will follow the pelvic curve as the head descends;

(10) *no attempt is made to rotate the head*; spontaneous rotation often occurs very late when the head is climbing the perineum just prior to delivery;

(11) an episiotomy is generally required; if the initial direction of traction is very posterior, the episiotomy may need to be carried out before traction commences;

(12) the cup is removed on delivery of the baby's head.

> If there is any possibility of borderline cephalo-pelvic disproportion, it will be safer to conduct the delivery as a 'trial of ventouse' in theatre.

The woman must be warned in advance about the chignon which will always result after a successful ventouse delivery. She must be strongly reassured that this is an entirely normal feature of her delivery and will disappear rapidly. Otherwise the unexpected sight of the chignon can be terrifying.

Failed ventouse delivery

If delivery is not imminent within four good contractions/traction episodes, cephalo-pelvic disproportion must be considered to be the cause. Prolonged attempts at traction can considerably traumatize the scalp and lead to sloughing of skin over the chignon.

Other reasons for failed ventouse are an incorrect line of pull during traction which probably leads to detachment of the cup, incorrect application of the cup in a too anterior position, inclusion of vaginal wall or cervix between the cup and scalp, and faulty equipment, especially a pump fault. If the cup does come off the scalp, it can be reapplied one more time over the chignon and suction re-established for a final attempt at delivery.

Caesarean section

Caesarean section may be planned antenatally as an elective procedure for maternal or fetal interests. The need for abdominal delivery may also arise as an emergency either antenatally or, more commonly, in labour.

In 1990, the Caesarean section rate in England and Wales was 12 per cent. The rate is rising, most probably through fear of litigation. It must be remembered that a Caesarean section is not without its consequences and has implications for future pregnancies. It should, therefore, not be undertaken without adequate indication. Caesarean section persistently features as a significant cause of maternal death. In the most recent Report on Confidential Enquiries into Maternal Deaths in the UK (1988–90) there were 91 maternal deaths following delivery by Caesarean section. Excluding the 12 'peri-mortem' operations where the terminally ill mother was receiving cardiopulmonary support, and the 8 post-mortem sections, there were 57 direct deaths, 18 indirect, and four fortuitous deaths. Hypertensive disorders (18 per cent), pulmonary embolism (14 per cent), and haemorrhage (12 per cent) were classified as the major causes of direct death.

In 21 cases there were avoidable factors linked to substandard care. These included inadequate postoperative recovery facilities, inappropriate delegation to inexperienced staff, and inadequate consultant involvement.

Indications for Caesarean section

ELECTIVE CAESAREAN SECTION

Maternal indications:
- two or more previous Caesarean sections
- when 'trial of scar' after one Caesarean section is contraindicated due to a recurring problem or to an additional problem arising in the subsequent pregnancy
- previous classical Caesarean section
- successful previous surgery for stress incontinence or fistula
- elderly primigravida plus an additional obstetric or medical problem
- certain cases of medical problems (diabetes, hypertension).

Fetal indications:
- some cases of IUGR
- higher order pregnancy (three or more).

Combined maternal and fetal indications:
- cephalo-pelvic disproportion (CPD)
- major degree of placenta praevia
- grim past obstetric history with no living children
- premium pregnancy (e.g. IVF) plus any significant problem
- certain malpresentations.

EMERGENCY CAESAREAN SECTION

Maternal indications:
- failure to progress in labour.

Fetal indications:
- fetal distress before or during the first stage of labour
- cord prolapse before or during the first stage of labour
- very preterm labour to deliver in the best condition
- failure to progress during a breech labour
- transverse lie in labour
- persistent brow presentation in labour
- antepartum haemorrhage
- premium pregnancy plus any significant problem arising in labour.

Combined maternal and fetal indications:
- failed 'trial of labour'
- failed 'trial of scar'
- failed 'trial of forceps or ventouse'.

For elective surgery, there is time to discuss the method of anaesthesia. Epidural or spinal block have much to recommend their use. The woman and her partner are able to share one of the most remarkable experiences of their lives. When it is known in advance that opening the abdomen is is likely to be difficult or take longer than usual because of dense scar tissue from previous operations, an epidural is ideal as it avoids exposing the baby to a prolonged general anaesthetic before delivery. The anaesthetist should see the woman preoperatively to answer any questions she may have and to allay any understandable fears. It is especially important to reassure her, if she has decided upon regional analgesia, that if at any stage during the delivery she should experience undue discomfort, either sedation or even general anaesthesia will be given. It is rare to find a couple who regret their decision to avoid a general anaesthetic. The epidural may also be used for postoperative pain relief.

NEVER force a woman into having her Caesarean section under regional block.

There are two situations where an epidural Caesarean section is not to be recommended. The first is an elective Caesarean section for a major degree of anterior placenta praevia. Considerable speed and dexterity is required to either deflect the placenta or deliver the baby through the placenta. In addition to this, the amount of blood loss can only be terrifying to a conscious patient, let alone her partner! Secondly, when an emergency Caesarean section is required to deliver the baby urgently, there is no place for first giving an epidural. A general anaesthetic will permit delivery with far greater speed. It can occasionally happen that a woman has a working epidural in labour and sudden dramatic fetal distress occurs. An epidural in such circumstances would probably require additional 'topping up' first and simply does not allow the surgeon to deliver the baby with adequate speed; a general anaesthetic in addition to the epidural is advisable.

It must be stressed that a Caesarean section under regional ananlgesia is not a procedure to be undertaken by an inexperienced surgeon. Surgical skills must be developed, under supervision, on the unconscious patient!

Elective Caesarean sections are generally performed at 38–39 weeks. A full blood count and at least a grouping and save serum is carried out. When it is known that the operation is likely to be haemorrhagic, as in placenta praevia cases, or difficult, as in repeat Caesarean sections, cross-matching of 2 units of blood is advisable. A consent form is signed. A supra-pubic shave is performed. The bladder is catheterized and the catheter is then left to drain into a pad so that the bladder remains empty during the course of the operation. The anaesthetist and paediatrician are informed.

Anaesthetic precautions and the use H_2-receptor blocking drugs have already discussed (p. 169). However, ranitidine may not always be effective in increasing the pH of the gastric contents. It is, therefore, recommended that during surgery, gastric aspiration should be performed to reduce the risk of postoperative aspiration and inhalation.

The Association of Anaesthetists have recommended the routine use of a CO_2 analyser which will show the presence of CO_2 in expired air. This is the only certain method of ensuring that the endotracheal tube is actually in the trachea. Monitoring by pulse oximeter throughout the operation is now standard routine practice.

The abdominal incision for Caesarean section is either a vertical sub-umbilical incision or a supra-pubic curved transverse (Pfannenstiel) incision.

The advantages of the *vertical incision* are speed, increased accessibility, and room to manoeuvre. These advantages can become very apparent if there is a very dense and fibrous transverse scar to reincise in the emergency situation. The disadvantages of the vertical incision are its general unsightliness and the inherent weakness of such scars where all the layers are repaired in a vertical direction.

The advantages of a *Pfannenstiel incision* are its preference by patients because it is aesthetically more pleasing in appearance and its general strength as the skin and rectus sheath layers are transverse to the peritoneal layer. The disadvantages are the increased skill required to open the abdomen, the increased risk of wound haematoma, and the increased time taken to deliver the baby. However, the Pfannenstiel incision is the standard incision taught to all aspiring obstetricians and gynaecologists, and undue difficulty should not arise except in repeat operations through the same scar. Haemostasis at the time of closure of the abdomen and wound drainage do much to reduce the risks of haematoma. Speed increases with experience. In the emergency situation there is no reason why the baby should not be delivered within 90 seconds.

Regardless of the direction of the skin incision, the uterine incision is either vertical (classical) or transverse in the lower segment of the uterus (Fig. 7.8).

The **classical Caesarean section** has limited use in modern obstetrics. The chief indications are, transverse lie in labour, very preterm operations when the lower segment has not yet formed and certain cases of major degrees of anterior placenta praevia, usually in combination with sterilization of the mother. The only advantages of the classical operation are dramatically increased accessibility and operative speed. Its very major disadvantage is that the vertical uterine scar in the upper segment does not heal so well owing to the involution of the uterus disturbing and possibly disrupting the healing process. As a result, there is a greater risk of antenatal scar dehiscence and uterine rupture in a subsequent

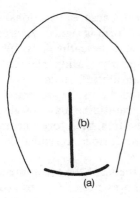

Fig. 7.8   Caesarean section incision in the uterus; (a) transverse lower segment incision; (b) vertical 'classical' upper segment incision.

labour. To reduce the chances of dehiscence, it is essential to close the vertical uterine incison with interrupted sutures, as a continuous suture will lossen as the uterus involutes. The implication of a classical Caesarean section is that all subsequent deliveries *must* be via the abdominal route.

The **lower segment Caesarean section** is the standard approach for the vast majority of abdominal deliveries. As the lower segment of the uterus remains relatively stable during the involution process of the uterus postnatally, healing is improved and the chances of uterine scar dehiscence are small. Because the uterine scar is reperitonealized, there is reduced risk of adhesion formation. The disadvantages of the lower segment approach are the increased skill required, the increased risk of the incision extending and involving the uterine artery, and the proximity of the bladder (and therefore increased risk of trauma to that organ).

If a general anaesthetic is to be given, the patient should not be anaesthetized until the abdomen has been cleaned and draped. This will significantly reduce the anaesthetic induction/delivery interval as the abdominal incision can be made almost immediately after intubation has been achieved.

Operative speed is important with regard to the incision/delivery interval. This can only be achieved with experience. There is no need to diathermy blood vessels on opening the abdominal wall. If left until the time of closure of the abdomen, most bleeding relating to the incision has stopped. The priority is to deliver the baby.

Operative skill can only be obtained by good teaching, good supervision, and experience.

Stages in lower segment Caesarean section

(1) the patient is in a left lateral tilt to avoid caval compression; the fetal heart is checked; the abdomen is opened (see above); ensure that the incision is adequate if a repeat operation through scar tissue;

(2) the peritoneal cavity is opened and a Doyen retractor is inserted to expose the utero-vesical fold of peritoneum;

(3) the utero-vesical peritoneum is picked up and incised transversely; the bladder is *gently* deflected downwards to reveal the lower segment of the uterus;

(4) the position of the Doyen retractor is adjusted so that the bladder is retracted gently out of the operative field; the insertion of a 'stay' suture in the lower segment just below the planned uterine incision line takes only seconds to perform and can be most helpful in identifying the lower margin of the incision at the time of closure;

(5) the uterine incision is made transversely in the centre of the lower segment until the membranes are visible; this is then extended transversely by the operator's fingers;

(6) if still intact, the bulging membranes are ruptured; the operator inserts a hand to deliver the lower pole of the baby with the assistance of fundal pressure; Wrigley's forceps can at times be very helpful in delivering the baby's head through the uterine incision;

(7) give intravenous ergometrine 0.25 mg or syntocinon 5 units; as soon as the head is delivered the baby's airways can be cleared; the cord is divided between two clamps;

(8) the placenta is delivered manually ensuring that no cotyledons or membranes remain within the uterus;

(9) adequate drainage of lochia is ensured by introducing a finger through the cervix from above;

(10) the lateral angles are held and secured with sutures; the uterine incision is repaired in two layers using a continuous suture, the second layer burying the first;

(11) after haemostasis is achieved, the utero-vesical peritoneum is closed; blood and clot are removed; the tubes and ovaries are checked; the abdomen is closed in layers; consider drain to rectus sheath;

(12) the uterus is firmly compressed through the abdominal wall to ensure it is well contracted and to remove clot; the vagina is cleared of clot; the catheter is removed.

The difficult Caesarean section can be a nightmare even for the experienced operator. DO NOT HESITATE TO SEEK HELP, ideally *before* problems arise.

Post-mortem Caesarean section

Very occasionally, the obstetrician will be asked to consider emergency delivery of the baby in a dead or dying woman. Success is only likely in the case of a patient who is being kept alive on a life support system. Consent should be sought from the relatives. A classical operation is performed and carried out with the full care normally given to a patient who is going to survive the procedure.

Symphysiotomy

There are many parts of the world where symphysiotomy is a safer procedure for the woman than Caesarean section, especially with regard to a subsequent labour. There are few indications for carrying out this operation in Western communities where there is easy access to Caesarean section. As a result, few obstetricians have experience of the procedure.

The chief indication for carrying out symphysiotomy is an outlet contracture of the pelvis recognized only late in labour. Symphysiotomy may also be indicated if outlet contraction is found in a breech labour when the baby is already delivered to the neck and still alive and well. The advantage of symphysiotomy is that a 2–3 cm increase in the transverse diameter of the outlet is obtained with widening of the sub-pubic angle. In a subsequent labour the symphysis readily opens to permit vaginal delivery.

The symphysis pubis is infiltrated with local anaesthetic. A pudendal block or perineal infiltration is also given. The bladder is catheterized and the catheter is used to manipulate the urethra and hold it to one side, away from the line of incision. The patient's legs are held by two assistants instead of lithotomy stirrups, as this allows for greater control of the degree of separation of the symphysis and significantly reduces the risk of soft tissue damage during that process.

The symphysiotomy is performed using either a 'closed' or 'open' method. For the 'closed' method, a solid scalpel is required, an instrument that probably does not feature on many UK labour wards. An incision is made at the upper border of the symphysis. The scalpel is inserted so that the blade lies flat against the anterior aspect of the symphysis pubis. The scalpel is then turned through 90 degrees so that the cutting edge is against the symphysis. As the incision is made through the fibres of the symphysis, the operator can assess the degree of separation of the fibres of the joint by holding the urethra to one side with the assistance of the indwelling catheter. The two assistants who are supporting the legs apply pressure to the trochanters and slightly abduct the legs at the direction of the operator. No more than 3 cm separation is sought. In the 'open' method, the mons pubis is incised. The symphysis is opened from behind in a forwards direction.

Once the symphysiotomy has been performed, the ventouse is most commonly used to complete the delivery. Following delivery, the patient's upper thighs are strapped together to provide support to the pelvis. She is not allowed to attempt walking for 4 days. The bladder may require an indwelling catheter as there is usually considerable oedema around the urethra which can result in retention of urine.

Additional labour ward emergencies

Shoulder dystocia

The baby's head is the widest fetal structure to pass through the mother's pelvis. If the baby is postmature or very large at term, the shoulders may obstruct further delivery after delivery of the head. If the baby is not delivered promptly, asphyxia and death will result.

Of the congenital abnormalities, the undiagnosed case of postmature anencephaly will most commonly be complicated by shoulder dystocia. A very distended fetal abdomen from ascites may also trap the fetus after delivery of the head.

Potential cases of shoulder dystocia can often be recognized antenatally. If vaginal delivery is planned, the notes should be clearly signalled to **'BEWARE SHOULDER DYSTOCIA!'**

The woman who had a previous large baby where there was difficulty in delivering the shoulders is likely to run into the same problem again. In such circumstances there is a good case for considering an elective Caesarean section. All postmature large babies are at risk. Delay in the second stage of labour in this situation is a warning of further trouble to come after delivery of the head.

If shoulder dystocia is anticipated, it is essential that an experienced obstetrician is available at the time of delivery.

Shoulder dystocia can be recognized by the experienced obstetrician on sight. Characteristically, once delivered, the large baby's head appears to be 'hugged into the perineum'. Attempts to deliver the baby in the normal manner fail and the head generally remains immobile.

DO NOT WASTE TIME. THIS IS AN OBSTETRIC EMERGENCY.
(Although it is easy to say, don't panic either!)

The patient should immediately be placed into the lithotomy position. A vaginal examination can be difficult but it should be possible to determine the plane of the shoulders. If an episiotomy has not been done then a generous one is performed taking care to guard the baby's neck. During maternal effort, the head, which is first restituted on the neck in line with the shoulders, is then drawn down towards the floor with the assistance of supra-pubic pressure over the anterior shoulder and fundal pressure applied by two assistants. This is usually successful in achieving delivery of the anterior shoulder, and the posterior shoulder should follow without difficulty.

If this should fail, the operator inserts a finger into each axilla and rather like Løvset's manoeuvre, rotates the baby's back so that it passes beneath the symphysis through 180 degrees. This brings the posterior shoulder into an anterior position under the symphysis and allows it to be delivered.

If this too should fail, the operator inserts a hand along the hollow of the sacrum and locates the posterior arm. Backward pressure against the elbow joint enables the forearm to be reached which is then drawn across the baby's chest and can be delivered. This should significantly reduce the transverse diameter across the shoulders and allow the delivery of the anterior shoulder to follow. In the presence of a really large baby this can be an extremely difficult manoeuvre. It is most helpful if an assistant applies traction to the head, but in an upward direction, while the posterior arm is being delivered.

Cleidotomy to deliberately fracture the clavicles is generally reserved for babies that are already dead, have a congenital abnormality, or as the very last resort. Should fetal ascites be present, the abdomen can be decompressed with a long needle.

Cord prolapse

There are several clinical situations where the risk of cord prolapse is significantly increased when the membranes rupture:

unstable lie after 38 weeks: if the lie is other than longitudinal, there will be no presenting part to fit into the pelvis if the membranes rupture;

polyhydramnios: the cord may be washed down with the gush of liquor;

cord presentation: the cord will definitely prolapse if it still presents at the time of membrane rupture;

flexed breech and footling breech presentations: poorly fitting presenting parts when compared to the extended breech;

amniotomy with a high presenting part: to be avoided unless in theatre with immediate access to Caesarean section.

In cases of unstable lie after 38 weeks and tense polyhydramnios, the woman should be admitted to hospital so that she is in the safest environment should spontaneous rupture of the membranes occur. Although this gives no guarantee of fetal survival should the cord prolapse, even in hospital, there will at least be a greater chance of a successful outcome. A cord prolapse in the home will generally imply loss of the baby. In such cases, as long as placenta praevia has been excluded, trained midwifery staff should be instructed to carry out an immediate vaginal examination to exclude cord prolapse in the event of spontaneous membrane rupture.

When the cord is presenting, it will definitely prolapse into the vagina upon rupture of the membranes. An emergency Caesarean section is the only safe option if this risk is to be avoided. It is also safer to deliver a footling breech by elective Caesarean section.

Cord prolapse may be diagnosed on vaginal examination or the cord may present outside the vagina. Cord prolapse is an indication for immediate delivery of the baby by the speediest route, as long as the baby is still alive. Generally this means immediate Caesarean section. If the cord has prolapsed outside the vulva it must be gently replaced into the vagina as the difference between the air and body temperatures can cause umbilical vessel spasm. Even handling the cord can have the same effect. The presenting part of the baby should be pushed gently upwards by the examining fingers *and held in that position* so that there is no direct pressure on the cord. Although seemingly undignified, the vaginal manipulation is continued while the patient is placed into the knee–chest position en route to the operating theatre. The fingers in the vagina are only removed at the moment of delivery.

If the cervix is fully dilated, vaginal delivery can be undertaken. A forceps delivery is performed for cephalic presentations. If the presentation is breech, a breech extraction can be carried out by an experienced operator, but only in the multiparous patient when all the circumstances are otherwise favourable.

If the cord has stopped pulsating, the baby will be dead. Vaginal delivery is achieved in the majority of cases.

Uterine rupture

Most cases of uterine rupture are associated with a previous Caesarean section scar, especially a classical scar. Scar rupture is associated with the poor selection of patients for a subsequent attempt at a vaginal delivery and the injudicious use of oxytocin. Care should be taken if vaginal prostaglandin is to be used to 'ripen' the cervix. The 'softening' effect of the prostaglandins on the cervix can also affect the scar.

Uterine rupture may also occur spontaneously without the presence of a uterine scar. It most commonly occurs in women of high parity where obstructed labour may arise due to cephalo-pelvic disproportion and malpresentations. Oxytocin unwisely given to the 'grand multip' can rupture the uterus even on a low-dose infusion regimen. Uterine rupture may also result from traumatic instrumental deliveries (including ventouse as well as forceps) and intrauterine manipulations. Cervical stenosis from previous cervical surgery can obstruct labour, the cervix becoming paper-thin with a 'pin-hole' os, until the stenotic ring either rapidly dilates or tears, extending up into the lower segment of the uterus.

Signs of uterine rupture

- maternal tachycardia
- severe fetal distress or sudden intrauterine death
- change in uterine shape due to a broad ligament haematoma or fetus delivered through rupture site
- change in the presenting part
- increased ease in palpating fetal parts
- vaginal bleeding varying from slight to torrential
- haematuria
- labour stops
- if rupture occurs late in the second stage, after the baby is delivered, *shortening* of the cord may be noted due to the placenta being extruded through the rupture site
- maternal collapse.

While the diagnosis may be obvious from the presenting signs, this is not always the case. The rupture of a previous section scar may be completely pain-free, the only sign being maternal tachycardia. When abdominal pain is present, it may be minimal or severe and described as 'bursting'. In such cases pain may be felt even through an effective epidural block. An epidural is, therefore, not contraindicated in a 'trial of scar' as it will not mask the pain of a ruptured uterus should pain be a significant feature.

Uterine rupture must be considered in all cases of maternal collapse.

In the collapsed patient, resuscitation is an urgent matter. Blood must be ordered in realistic volumes of 4–6 units. Examination under anaesthesia will confirm the diagnosis, and laparotomy is performed. At laparotomy, the baby (which is invariably dead) and the placenta may be lying outside the uterus. There may be a considerable quantity of blood in the peritoneal cavity.

The majority of even severe uterine ruptures can be repaired. The decision as to whether or not to repair the uterus or carry out a hysterectomy *must* be made by a consultant obstetrician.

The woman's condition, her age, parity, and her desire to increase the size of her family, are all factors which will influence the final decision. At the end of the operation the pelvis must be drained. Antibiotic therapy commenced during the operation is wise as postoperative infection is otherwise inevitable.

If the uterus has been successfully repaired, this is not a bar to future pregnancies. Elective Caesarean section, possibly classical to avoid complex repair work in the lower segment, would be indicated at 36–38 weeks.

In the Report on Confidential Enquiries into Maternal Deaths in the UK (1988–90) there were two direct deaths due to spontaneous uterine rupture. In the first case, a classical Caesarean section scar ruptured at term before the onset of labour with massive intra-abdominal haemorrhage. This very obese patient had a long psychiatric history, was not known to be pregnant, and had had no antenatal care. In the second case, a 'grand multip' with a severe abruptio placentae leading to intrauterine death at 37 weeks, had labour induced by amniotomy and low-dosage syntocinon. Following vaginal delivery, persistent postpartum haemorrhage and DIC led to laparotomy which revealed the rupture. At hysterectomy recurrent ventricular fibrillation led to death. Care was considered to be substandard in both cases.

> The use of syntocinon infusions in patients of high multiparity is always potentially dangerous.

When deaths do occur due to uterine rupture, the most significant factor is substandard care in labour. This is largely due to the inexperience of the doctors in charge, delayed diagnosis, inadequate resuscitation, and failure to call soon enough for senior experienced assistance.

Inversion of the uterus

The aim of controlled cord traction is to prevent the fundus of the contracted uterus from 'following' the placenta into the vagina. The rare complication of uterine inversion is invariably due to attempts made to deliver the placenta when the uterus is not contracted and before there are signs of placental separation. In these cases the placental site tends to be at the fundus. Occasionally inversion is associated with a morbid adherence of the placenta to the uterus (placenta accreta) and a very short cord.

The signs of uterine inversion are the disappearance of the uterus from the abdomen and either seeing or feeling the uterus in the vagina.

Immediate replacement of the uterus is essential to avoid maternal shock, haemorrhage, and even death.

Do not attempt to remove the placenta first. Speed in replacing the uterus is vital.

If there is any delay, a tight constriction ring will form preventing manual replacement of the uterus. In this situation, intravenous uterine relaxants such as ritodrine may be helpful. Halothane administered by the anaesthetist should also produce sufficient relaxation of the constriction ring to allow replacement of the uterus. Successful replacement may also be achieved using hydrostatic pressure. The vagina is filled with 2 litres of warm saline via a cystoscopy tube while the labia are kept closed by the forearm of the operator or the hands of an assistant. The build-up of intravaginal pressure replaces the uterus into the abdomen through the constriction ring. Only after successful replacement of the uterus is any further attempt made to deliver the placenta. The uterus is kept well-contracted with a syntocinon infusion over the next 4 hours.

Amniotic fluid embolism

This (fortunately) rare and generally fatal condition arises in situations where there is an increased intrauterine pressure able to force amniotic fluid into the maternal circulation. The condition is associated with high parity, women over the age of 35 years, precipitate labour, excessive oxytocin dosage (especially single-bolus dose of syntocinon or syntometrine), hypertonic uterine activity, overdistension of the uterus as in polyhydramnios, uterine rupture, and disseminated intravascular coagulation.

In the Report on Confidential Enquiries into Maternal Deaths in the UK (1988–90), there were 11 proven deaths due to amniotic fluid embolism. Although all of the patients were over 25 years of age, none were of high parity. Seven of the patients had labour induced and one had an elective Caesarean section. Eight were eventually delivered by Caesarean section. Three of the 6 emergency Caesarean sections were for maternal collapse, the remaining 3 for fetal distress. Four patients had a postpartum haemorrhage.

Amniotic fluid embolism must be suspected in all cases of sudden collapse in labour or the immediate postpartum period.

The characteristic features of amniotic fluid embolism include sudden acute dyspnoea with signs of cardiovascular collapse. Death can occur with extraordinary speed, the condition being fatal in all but a minority of patients. In those who survive for more than the first 30 minutes, disseminated intravascular coagulopathy (DIC) develops. Profuse postpartum haemorrhage occurs which will not respond to normal measures.

Essentially, the treatment problem that presents is that of a pulmonary embolism with cardiopulmonary collapse and torrential vaginal haemorrhage due to DIC. Survival of the patient depends on the speed of initial resuscitation and subsequent management between the intensive care unit and haematology department.

Management of amniotic fluid embolism

(1) oxygen is initially given by face mask until intubated by the anaesthetist and then continued by intermittent positive pressure ventilation;

(2) correction of acidosis and maintenance of the circulation is essential; care must be taken not to overload the circulation and a central venous pressure line is invaluable;

(3) high doses of intravenous hydrocortisone (1 g 1–2 hourly) are indicated;

(4) the DIC must be corrected and controlled; while an urgent clotting screen is requested, heparin 5000 units is given intravenously; fresh frozen plasma is also required;

(5) vaginal haemorrhage must be controlled by stimulating the uterus to contract.

The confirmation of the diagnosis of amniotic fluid embolism has until recently only been possible at post-mortem. It is now possible to find fetal squames and hair in blood aspirated from the pulmonary artery using a Swan–Ganz catheter, or even in maternal sputum.

Problems in the third stage of labour

Postpartum haemorrhage (PPH)

Postpartum haemorhage is defined as vaginal blood loss of 500 ml or more occurring after delivery of the baby. Primary PPH occurs within 24 hours of delivery of the baby. Secondary PPH occurs within 6 weeks of delivery (see p. 258).

Primary PPH may therefore occur whether or not the placenta has been delivered.

The chief cause of postpartum haemorrhage is poor uterine retraction.

Retraction is the ability of uterine muscle to maintain tone during the relaxation phase between contractions. This is particularly important at the placental site. If the uterus is atonic for any reason, its ability to retract will be reduced. The upper segment of the uterus with its increased musculature is able to retract more than the lower segment. If the placenta is encroaching onto the lower segment of the uterus, placental site retraction is poor and PPH is commoner.

Predisposing factors causing primary PPH

Reduced retraction leading to atony

increasing maternal age: even among women of low parity, increased maternal age increase the risks of haemorrhage

grand multiparity precipitate labour; poor health and anaemia increase risks of PPH;

overdistended uterus:
multiple pregnancy; the placental site is larger and more likely to encroach upon the lower segment where retraction is poor *polyhydramnios;*

APH (placenta praevia and abruptio placentae)

prolonged labour: poor uterine contractions in the first stage of labour may continue into the second and third stages

precipitate labour other than grand multipara

retained placental tissue

past history of PPH

full bladder can prevent the uterus from contracting effectively;

fibroids.

Utero-vaginal trauma
vaginal and cervical tears, episiotomy: delay in repair can lead to exsanguination

uterine rupture

inversion of the uterus.

Coagulopathy
disseminated intravascular coagulation (DIC)

amniotic fluid embolism;

congenital coagulation defects (such as factor VIII deficiency).

PPH will occur in up to 2 per cent of deliveries. In the Report on Confidential Enquiries into Maternal Deaths (1988–90) there were 11 deaths directly caused by PPH without preceeding APH. Four of the PPHs followed Caesarean section, 3 were associated with forceps delivery, and 1 with ventouse delivery. DIC complicated 4 cases. Care was judged to be substandard in 8 of the 11 deaths due to PPH.

There is evidence to suggest that obstetricians are becoming less vigilant and less experienced than in the past when it comes to treating a life-threatening haemorrhage. Inappropriate delegation of Caesarean section and difficult vaginal tear repairs to junior staff, failure to recognize DIC, and inadequate postnatal observation were all at fault.

Death from PPH is avoidable in the majority of cases.

(1) high-risk patients must be booked into a consultant unit with intensive care facilities;

(2) experienced medical and midwifery staff must be present;

(3) the third stage of labour must be managed correctly, including the routine use of oxytocic drugs;

(4) anaemia should be corrected *before* labour; if not, cross-matched blood must be available during labour.

Management of PPH

Beware the persistent trickle of blood in the third stage of labour, especially in patients who have predisposing factors for PPH. Awareness of the potential problems is vital. There are few things in obstetrics more terrifying than torrential haemorrhage. In the event of PPH occuring in the patient's home or in a non-consultant unit, the 'flying squad' or paramedic ambulance service must be called to resuscitate. The role of the 'flying squad' is to resuscitate the patient before transferring to the consultant unit.

A significant PPH cannot be managed single-handed. SEEK HELP IMMEDIATELY.

Prolonged hypotension from haemorrhage runs the risk of pituitary necrosis (Sheehan's syndrome) which is suspected later if there is failure of lactation and amenorrhoea.

When a major PPH occurs, the patient's very survival will depend upon an experienced team of obstetrician, midwife, anaesthetist, haematologist, and on-site intensive care facilities. THIS MUST NOT BE DEALT WITH AT A JUNIOR LEVEL. Junior staff sometimes complain that they meet with obstruction from a blood transfusion technician or even portering services. **Call in the consultant staff.**

Management of PPH

(1) If the uterus is atonic, **'rub-up' a contraction** by massaging the fundus of the uterus;

(2) **deliver the placenta if undelivered;**

(3) **give intravenous ergometrine 0.5 mg** (there are no contraindications in the haemorrhaging patient);

(4) if this controls the haemorrhage give **syntocinon** 40 units in 500 ml of 5% dextrose 4-hourly;

(5) in major PPH, **set up two intravenous infusion lines;** a **central venous pressure (CVP) line** is essential to accurately control the volume of blood to be replaced;

(6) if the uterus remains atonic, a **myometrial injection of prostaglandin F_2 alpha 1 mg** should be administered (unless the patient is asthmatic);

(7) **urgently cross-match realistic volumes of blood;** in a major PPH request 6 units of **whole blood;** while awaiting the blood, the use of volume expanders such as haemacel will be necessary;

(8) an **emergency coagulation profile** will take time; meanwhile, check clotting by placing 5 ml of blood in a glass tube and invert periodically; a clotting time of more than 12 minutes indicates a coagulopathy; in very severe PPH, this is an indication for giving **fresh frozen plasma;**

(9) **replace blood rapidly;** use a **compression cuff** on the blood bag; use **blood-warming equipment;** in dire emergency use **uncross-matched O-negative** blood

(10) **check the placenta for completeness;**

(11) **ensure that the bladder is empty;**

(12) **bimanual compression** of the uterus can be helpful;

(13) **suspect genital tract trauma** if heavy bleeding occurs in spite of the uterus being well contracted;

(14) **examination under anaesthesia** is required to adequately explore the uterine cavity for retained placental cotyledons and clot; vaginal, cervical, and uterine trauma can be assessed and repaired;

(15) **hot intrauterine douching** with saline via intravenous drip tubing can stimulated the uterus to contract;

(16) **intrauterine packing** is difficult to perform but may occasionally succeed in controlling blood loss;

(17) **direct aortic compression** can be life-saving during **ligation of internal iliac arteries** or **hysterectomy.**

Treatment and investigation go hand in hand. The principles of the management of haemorrhage are to locate and control the source of bleeding, replace the blood lost, and correct shock. In the presence of haemorrhage all other rules are broken. **THE PATIENT WILL OTHERWISE DIE**.

Retained placenta

If the placenta is not delivered within 20 minutes, seek help.

Manual removal of placenta

(1) The patient is placed into lithotomy and the perineum is cleaned and draped; the bladder is catheterized;

(2) a vaginal examination is performed, gently introducing the entire hand into the vagina;

(3) the cervix is now slowly but firmly dilated with the tips of the examining fingers; the uterus is stabilized with the external hand against the abdominal wall;

(4) the fingers now follow the cord (if it is still attached to the placenta) to its insertion; the whole of the examining hand is now in the uterus;

(5) while continuing to stabilize the uterus with the external hand, the hand in the uterus locates the placental edge; holding the fingers firmly together in one plane, the hand is used as a slice to separate the placenta from its site of attachment;

(6) the external hand is able to guide the fundus of the uterus onto the examining hand and so assist in separating the placenta and reducing the risk of perforating the uterus;

(7) only when the placenta has been completely separated from the uterine wall is it removed; piecemeal removal increases the risk of haemorrhage;

(8) the cavity is now explored carefully to ensure that there are no placental cotyledons left behind;

(9) a syntocinon infusion is set up (40 units in 500 ml of 5 per cent dextrose) to run over the next 4 hours;

(10) appropriate antibiotic therapy is given in view of the extensive intrauterine manipulation.

Under these circumstances, it is always worth while to carry out a vaginal examination. If the placenta is found to be partly in the vagina with the cervix clamped down on to it, direct traction of the vaginal portion of placenta combined with maternal effort should be successful. If the placenta is trapped above the cervix, a further attempt at gentle, controlled cord traction with maternal effort is reasonable. If this fails, or there is sudden 'give' in the cord, indicating that it is about to tear, a **manual removal of placenta** must be carried out. If a retained placenta occurs away from the consultant unit, the 'flying squad' must be called.

Blood is sent for cross-matching. An anaesthetic is necessary, a good epiduaral being adequate. The aim of the manoeuvre is explained to the patient.

Very occasionally, the placenta is found to be morbidly adherent to the uterine wall. Complete separation of the placenta accreta is impossible and brisk haemorrhage follows. This situation can occasionally be found at Caesarean section. Firm packing of the uterine cavity may control blood loss, but may only be a delaying manoeuvre before having to resort to hysterectomy.

HELLP syndrome

This syndrome is characterized by *H*aemolysis, *E*levated *L*iver enzymes, and *L*ow *P*latelets. Women who subsequently develop HELLP are frequently admitted complaining of epigastric pain. They may be hypertensive at admission. Proteinuria is usually a feature. They may initially be regarded as having severe pregnancy-induced hypertension.

After delivery, the patient's condition worsens. The epigastric pain becomes severe. Hypertension usually develops. Oliguria and proteinuria may be observed. Eclampsia may occur.

> Be aware of HELLP. Always investigate epigastric pain, even in the absence of hypertension.

Thrombocytopenia develops with a drop in the platelet count to below 100 and often below 50×10^9. Liver function tests show a marked increase in liver enzymes, particularly gamma glutamyl transferase (GGT), alanine transaminase (ALT), aspartate transaminase (AST), and lactic dehydrogenase (LDH).

> Beware pregnancy-induced hypertension and thrombocytopenia.

These patients require high-dependency care when only moderately affected. Intensive care facilities and even dialysis are necessary in severe cases.

Flying squad

The role of the obstetric 'flying squad' has changed over the last 15 years with the reduction in domiciliary deliveries and the closure of many of the smaller peripheral GP maternity units. The call-out rate will vary in different parts of the country but ranges between 1 and 2 per 1000 deliveries.

A recent survey (Royal College of Midwives 1989) showed that the majority of calls were indicated for haemorrhage requiring possible resuscitation (78.5 per cent), specialist obstetric care including preterm labour, breech presentation, fetal distress, and cord prolapse (16.4 per cent), and eclampsia (5.1 per cent).

The major role of the 'flying squad' has been to resuscitate and transfer to the consultant unit. Operative delivery such as forceps or manual removal of a retained placenta is now rarely performed by the squad. It is, therefore, likely that with the increasing emergence of paramedic ambulance teams, such teams will in future be called out primarily to assess and resuscitate. This will have the advantage of not depleting the base hospital of trained staff required for the care of high-risk in-patients. There will always remain the facility for the midwife, GP, or paramedic team to call for the assistance of specialist obstetric care (consultant or senior registrar).

8 The newborn baby

Neonatal resuscitation

Most babies are delivered in good condition and do not need to be resuscitated. But unexpected neonatal emergencies frequently occur.

> It is the responsibility of every midwife and all medical staff on the labour ward to be familiar with the resuscitation equipment and to develop the necessary skills to carry out the basic techniques of neonatal resuscitation.

There are certain clinical situations where it can be predicted that resuscitation may be necessary. The neonatal unit should be informed by the labour ward staff when there is likely to be any concern over fetal well-being. A paediatrician should be requested to attend these deliveries.

> *Paediatric attendance at delivery*
>
> - all major obstetric complications
> - intrauterine growth retardation
> - multiple pregnancies
> - preterm labour
> - fetal distress/heavily meconium-stained liquor
> - all operative deliveries apart from straightforward lift-out forceps deliveries
> - pyrexia in labour
> - the mother has received opiates within 3 hours of delivery.

At delivery, once the baby's nose *and* mouth have been delivered, the naso-pharynx can be aspirated by the attending midwife. Once delivered, the baby is dried, wrapped in a warmed blanket and, if all is well, handed to the mother.

The initial assessment of the newborn baby is by Apgar scoring (Fig. 8.1).

The Apgar score is assessed at intervals of 1 and 5 minutes after birth. Although the Apgar score gives a numerical evaluation of well-being, it is the assessments for respiration and the heart rate which are of particular importance and will indicate whether or not resuscitation will be required. If the score is

Apgar Score

Sign	Score		
	0	**1**	**2**
Heart rate	Absent	< 100	> 100
Respiratory effort	Absent	v. irregular	good/crying
Muscle tone	Limp	Some flexion	Active movement
Reflex response	Absent	Minimal	Normal
Colour	Blue or pale	Blue extremities	Completely pink

Fig. 8.1 Apgar Score.

between 8 and 10, there is usually no cause for concern. An Apgar score of less than 8 at 1 minute indicates hypoxia and the need for resuscitative measures.

The aims of resuscitation

- clear airways
- establish ventilation
- maintain warmth.

Only 50 per cent of the babies requiring intubation are predicted by an awareness of risk factors. This highlights the importance of labour ward staff being familiar with neonatal resuscitation techniques.

Neonatal resuscitation

(1) the nasopharynx is cleared by suction if not already performed during the delivery;

(2) if the baby does not gasp within 1 minute of delivery, this is an indication to give 100 per cent oxygen; if the baby has been born in an asphyxiated condition or is floppy with a heart rate of less than 100, there is nothing to be gained by delay — RESUSCITATE!

(3) This should be carried out on a resuscitation trolley where the baby is placed in a head-down tilt;

(4) if **meconium** is present at delivery, this must be cleared from the airways *before* ventilation is given (see below);

(5) in the absence of meconium, as long as the heart rate is over 100 per minute, oxygen is initially given by face mask so as to be available when a spontaneous gasp is taken;

(6) if apnoea continues, intermittent positive pressure ventiliation (IPPR) is performed using bag and face mask; the ventilation pressure must not be above 30 cm of water and each ventilation should be for less than 2 seconds;

(7) if the baby still does not breathe spontaneously, or the heart rate is less than 100 per minute, intubation and IPPR is given; ventilation is continued until the baby is in good condition and breathing spontaneously;

(8) when meconium is present at delivery, a laryngoscope is passed to visualize the glottis; if meconium is seen this is an indication for *immediate* intubation and suction before aspiration can occur; once clear of meconium, 100 per cent oxygen is given; even if the baby has already gasped and aspirated meconium, suction alone is usually adequate before giving oxygen; lavage with normal saline and suction are only necessary if the meconium is very tenacious;

(9) **babies lose heat rapidly**; the baby must be kept warm; (operating theatres can often be cold) resuscitation trolleys are fitted with a radiant heater;

(10) if there is no detectable heart beat, after intubation and IPPR with 100 per cent oxygen, **external cardiac massage** is carried out; five compressions are given out to the midsection of the sternum for every lung inflation; acidosis is corrected by giving bicarbonate (5 mmol per kg) via an umbilical vein catheter.

The condition of the baby and the length of time of resuscitation will determine whether or not the baby accompanies the mother to the postnatal ward or is observed on the neonatal unit.

The healthy baby will have an initial examination shortly after delivery. A routine examination is carried out by the paediatrician within 48 hours and often repeated just before discharge home.

First examination

> One in 30 babies will have a congenital abnormality which may be very minor, or occasionally major and even lethal.

The first examination is a general overview of the baby's external features to be able to reassure the parents that 'everything is all right' and to state the sex of the baby. It can occasionally be difficult to determine the sex. DO NOT GUESS. Instead, inform the parents that sexing a baby is not always possible from the appearance of the external genitalia at birth and that further examination will be necessary.

A Hollister cord clamp is applied close to the umbilicus and redundant cord is excised. If there is only a single umbilical artery, this is an indication for renal ultrasound to exclude a renal abnormality. The baby is weighed.

In cases of polyhydramnios, a suction tube should be passed into the baby's stomach to exclude oesophageal atresia. The rectal temperature is taken to exclude an imperforate anus.

Vitamin K

It has been routine to give all newborn babies an intramuscular injection of vitamin K as soon as possible after birth, as a prophylaxis against haemorrhagic disease of the newborn. There has recently been an apparent, and as yet unproven, association between prophylactic vitamin K and leukaemia later in life. However, a 1993 study using hospital records from Sweden concluded that there was no relationship between injected vitamin K and childhood cancer in the group of 1 384 424 babies studied. Balanced against this remote theoretical risk is the *known hazard* of a 1 in 1000 chance of a major gastrointestinal bleed and 1 in 5000 chance of a lethal intracranial haemorrhage if vitamin K is witheld. The problem as to whether or not to give vitamin K is only one for women who have elected to breast-feed their babies. Artificial feeds all contain vitamin K and these babies will automatically be protected from haemolytic disease. The very significant risks of declining vitamin K to the babies of breast-feeding mothers must be made clear.

Routine examination

This examination gives the paediatrician the opportunity of detecting any abnormalities that may have been missed shortly after birth. This should be carried out in the presence of the parents who, generally, greatly enjoy the guided tour of their baby's examination.

Routine examination of the baby

(1) **general inspection** to look for obvious abnormalities and to assess posture, movements, reflex, and alertness;

(2) **examination of the head:** palpation of fontanelles (? tense); measurement of head circumference;

(3) **check the eyes** for ability to follow movement, abnormalities, and infection;

(4) **inspect the face:** ? features suggesting chromosomal abnormality (Down's syndrome);

(5) **examine the mouth** (inspection and palpation) to exclude palate and other abnormalities;

(6) **palpate the neck** to exclude thyroid enlargement and sternomastoid tumour; ? webbing of the neck (Turner's);

(7) **check the heart** for murmurs; check peripheral pulses (absent femoral pulses = coarctation of aorta);

(8) **palpate the abdomen** (it is normal to feel the liver edge, kidneys, and even the spleen); the cord stump is checked to ensure that there is no infection present, and to exclude minor degrees of exomphalos;

(9) **check external genitalia** to ensure that in the male infant there is no hypospadias and the testicles have descended, and that in the female there is no labial fusion;

(10) **examine for congenital dislocation of the hips and for talipes;**

(11) **examine the back** as a small encephalocele can be missed.

Reassurance is given over any minor problem such as skin marking, conjunctival haemorrhage, breast enlargement (in both sexes), and vaginal discharge.

Should any significant problems be found, these must be referred to the relevant specialist before discharge from hospital.

Guthrie test

All babies should undergo routine mass screening for phenylketonuria and hypo-thyroidism. Some units are also carrying out routine screening for cystic fibrosis from the same heel prick sample, as well as anonymous HIV antibody screening to assess the prevalence of this condition.

The blood sample is taken after the baby has had 48 hours of an adequate protein diet, whether breast- or bottle-fed.

- **phenylketonuria** is screened by measuring phenylalanine, using a flurometric method which is not affected by antibiotics;
- **hypothyroidism** is diagnosed by assay of the thyroid stimulating hormone level;
- **cystic fibrosis** screening is by radio-immunoassay for immune reactive trypsin.

Jaundice

Jaundice is never apparent at birth as the mother excretes fetal unconjugated bilirubin. Most babies will develop very mild physiological jaundice until the liver is competent and mature enough to conjugate bilirubin. Jaundice is, therefore, a common feature among preterm babies. It is also virtually a normal finding among breast-fed babies, as breast milk is able to convert conjugated bilirubin excreted into the bowel back into the unconjugated form which is then absorbed. Physiological jaundice appears by the second day and has cleared by the tenth day. The baby is generally well. However, the preterm baby can develop very high levels of bilirubin. Unconjugated bilirubin is bound to albumin and if all the available albumin is bound, excess bilirubin can cross the 'blood–brain barrier', with the risk of brain damage due to kernicterus. Plasma bilirubin levels above 200 μmol/l require treatment. Apart from very preterm or ill babies (where lower levels apply) unconjugated bilirubin levels greater than 350 μmol/l are dangerous and risk brain damage. Babies with intrapartum hypoxia, infections (particularly urinary tract infections), and hypothyroidism are more likely to develop jaundice.

Jaundice will also occur if bilirubin production is increased.

Rarely, jaundice is found to be due to high levels of *conjugated* bilirubin. This will indicate an obstructive cause such as a congenital biliary atresia and hepatitis.

Factors which increase bilirubin production

Haemolysis
  rhesus iso-immunization
  ABO incompatibility
  glucose-6-phosphate dehydrogenase deficiency
  congenital spherocytosis
Bruising
  traumatic delivery
  cephalohaematoma

All babies with jaundice, especially if unwell or preterm, must be investigated.

Investigation of neonatal jaundice

- **blood group** (mother and baby)
- **full blood count** including reticulocyte count and differential white cell count
- **Coombs test**
- **serial unconjugated bilirubin level**
- if **infection** suspected:
    urine sample sent for culture
    throat swab
    umbilical swab
    stool culture
    blood culture
    lumbar puncture
    chest X-ray
- thyroid stimulating hormone (**Guthrie test**)

A bilirubin above 200 μmol/l is initially treated by phototherapy. Phototherapy utilizes the effects of the blue wavelengths of light and is extremely effective in breaking down unconjugated bilirubin. Owing to the brightness of the light, it is usual to cover the baby's eyes with patches. If the technique and aims of phototherapy are explained to the parents in advance, distress at the sight of their baby receiving treatment can be significantly reduced.

If the bilirubin level is above 350 μmol/l exchange transfusion may be necessary. This is usually only required when the jaundice is due to excessive haemolysis.

9   Perinatal and maternal death

Perinatal death

A perinatal death is one which occurs between the 24th week of gestation and the end of the first week after birth. It therefore includes all stillbirths and early neonatal deaths. The reason for grouping these deaths together is because their aetiology is often the same. The perinatal mortality rate is the number of such deaths per thousand total births (stillbirths and live births).

Until 1992, a stillbirth in the UK was defined as a baby that was born dead after the 28th week of gestation. The perinatal mortality rate under this definition was in the region of 10 per 1000 total births. As viability is now considered to be possible at 24 weeks, the additional 4 weeks of stillbirths between 24 and 28 weeks is included in the perinatal mortality rate, live births already being included. The effect of this will be to increase the UK perinatal mortality rate to probably between 10 and 12 per 1000 total births.

There is considerable variation between different maternity units, with the curious anomaly of the smaller units having better perinatal statistics. The reason for this is that very preterm labours tend to become *in utero* transfers to major units with intensive care neonatal facilities. The perinatal mortality of *in utero* transfers can be as high as 120 per 1000 total births with a 60–70 per cent Caesarean section rate.

Management of intrauterine death

Apart from an intrauterine death resulting from an obstetric emergency such as placental abruption, it is usually the woman who is the first to become concerned about the well-being of her baby. Worried about an absence or reduction of kicks, she contacts her midwife, GP, or the hospital directly. The silence of the fetal heart on auscultation is confirmed by ultrasound which fails to show any fetal heart movement or other fetal activity. When the scan is completed she should be seen by a senior member of the obstetric team on duty, ideally with her partner and a midwife in attendance. It is often the case that she is already aware that something is wrong, having quickly picked up the concern and silence of her attendants. She should be told simply and with great sympathy that her baby's heart has stopped beating and that the baby has died.

This confirmation of her worst fears is devastating. If she is without her partner he should be called to the hospital. Time must be made available to give at least preliminary answers to their questions, and especially to reassure them that

Causes of perinatal death

Congenital abnormalities
chromomal abnormalities
fetal abnormalities:
   neural tube defects
   anencephaly
   cardiac anomalies
   other lethal abnormalities

Low birth weight
intrauterine growth retardation:
   essential hypertension
   pregnancy-induced hypertension
   smoking
   infection (cytomegalovirus, toxoplasmosis, rubella)
preterm labour:
   uterine abnormalities
   cervical incompetence
   premature induction
   multiple pregnancy
   polyhydramnios
   premature spontaneous rupture of membranes
   infection (β-haemolytic streptococcus)

Hypoxia in labour
antepartum baemorrhage:
   abruptio placentae
   placenta praevia
cord accidents:
   cord prolapse
   true knot in cord
   major cord entanglement (tightly around neck several times)

Unexplained stillbirth
? antenatal hypoxia
? cord entanglement

Hypoxia postpartum
respiratory distress syndrome infection

Birth trauma
intracranial haemorrhage:
   breech delivery
   precipitate labour
   traumatic instrumental delivery
   undiagnosed cephalo-pelvic disproportion

the tragedy is not the result of anything that she has or has not done. It is usually only possible at this stage to state that final answers to their questions will *perhaps* only become clear after the baby has been delivered.

The immediate future plans of action are discussed. The majority of women do not enjoy the prospect of carrying a dead baby. Admission should be offered with a view to induction the following day. She may, however, prefer to return home and be in the comfort of her own environment and have the support of her family for a while before admission. She should not be allowed to go home alone.

Some units have a separate suite that can be offered to a couple within the maternity unit, where they may stay together before and after delivery. This is ideal as contact at this stage with other pregnant women is likely to be mutually distressing.

There are two important aims in the conduct of labour:

- it is essential that the induction should not fail
- the labour should be pain-free.

Cervical 'ripening' with prostaglandin pessaries may be necessary. The anaesthetist should see the patient and discuss the method of analgesia. A regional block is very suitable for many women. Others may prefer to know as little as possible of events and opt for sedation. Diamorphine 5 mg provides excellent sedation.

The woman's partner, or other family member of her choice, should be encouraged to stay with her throughout labour. Delivery is generally accomplished without difficulty but may require forceps. The couple will usually have already decided whether or not they wish to see and hold the baby at this stage. Even a very macerated baby with major abnormalities can be wrapped in such a way so as to reduce distress. Couples will never regret seeing their dead baby even if this is deferred initially, as by doing so, the baby is given an identity they can grieve over. Most obstetricians have experience of couples who bitterly regret *not* having seen their baby and subsequently find that the whole experience is like a bad dream and their grief is unfocused. The baby should always be photographed and the photographs kept in a sealed envelope in the notes. These pictures are often requested by the couple at a later date. They should be encouraged to name their child and also be given the opportunity of seeing a minister of their own religion.

The baby should be seen by the obstetric staff on duty and any abnormalities noted must be documented. It is very helpful if the duty paediatrician also examines the baby.

So as to be in a position to fully answer all queries, it is essential to do everything possible to obtain relevant screening material from the woman, baby, and placenta. The labour ward is not the ideal environment to discuss the question of post-mortem unless the couple raise this first. It is kinder to defer this discussion until the next day. The importance of post-mortem cannot be over-stressed but the parents must not be coerced into giving their consent for this. Indeed, it may be against their religious beliefs to do so.

Investigations after delivery of a stillborn baby

Maternal
- full blood count
- Kleihauer
- HbA^{1c}
- cervical swabs for culture
- liquor swabs for culture (if not obtained during labour, take swab from the baby's ear);
- in severe IUGR or hydropic baby, maternal serum is required for a full TORCH screen and parvovirus

Fetal
- fetal karyotype; axillary skin biopsy placed in a saline-filled sterile container and sent directly to cytogenetics or refrigerated overnight; a fetal blood sample from a cardiac puncture (5 ml in a lithium heparin bottle) is also sent to cytogenetics
- congenital infection is screened by a cardiac blood sample for TORCH screen and parvovirus
- viral culture from a throat swab
- medical photography should be taken, apart from any labour ward Polaroid snaps that have been taken for the couple
- full skeletal X-ray is required; this can be requested via the mortuary.

Placenta
- swabs are taken for culture and sensitivity
- full histological report is requested (the placenta may be placed in formalin).

After delivery the baby should be kept in the mortuary until the parents have had an opportunity to decide about post-mortem. They may even wish to see the baby again. The couple should return to their room in the hospital for the night.

The Stillbirth Certificate is signed and every assistance is given to reduce distress to the couple. If they do not wish to make private funeral arrangements for the baby, the hospital will carry this out on their behalf, free of charge. *It is important* to make it clear to them that the grave will not have a named headstone as it is a communal grave shared with other babies. Failure to clarify this can cause considerable anger and grief if the couple try at some later date to find their baby's grave.

Before leaving the hospital, the couple should be seen by their consultant. Further information may now be available as to the cause of the baby's death. Sufficient time must be given to answer their questions, to allay any guilt that might be felt and even anger against medical attendants for not having been able to save their baby.

'Why did it happen?' Unless there is an obvious cause of death such as abruptio placentae with a large retro-placental clot, a true knot in the cord, or a major congenital abnormality, it may not be possible to answer this question until after the post-mortem has been carried out. The couple should be warned that the post-mortem may fail to come to any conclusion and the stillbirth will then be 'unexplained'. This can be very difficult for them to come to terms with and an explanation of antenatal hypoxia will be necessary.

'Will it happen again?' They should be reassured that it is very rare for a woman to have recurrent stillbirths. However, there are certain congenital abnormalities that do have a recurrent risk such as neural tube defects and inherited disorders. The assistance of a clinical geneticist can be most helpful and patients will usually appreciate the opportunity of a referral for genetic counselling. Amniocentesis may be recommended in a future pregnancy. Advice regarding pre-conception folic acid (0.4 mg daily) continued for the first 12 weeks of pregnancy should be given. If hypertension featured in the pregnancy, the question of low-dose aspirin in a future pregnancy should be discussed. If she is a smoker, suggestions on how to stop smoking before the next pregnancy will be appropriate. Everything possible must be done so that she is tingling with health before becoming pregnant again.

'When can we try again?' The short answer to this question is 'when you feel ready to do so'. There should not be a statutory ruling of a 6-month or 1-year delay. However, they should be advised to wait until they really *do* feel ready. Some couples feel that they want to start another pregnancy as quickly as possible, as if in some way the new pregnancy will blot out their grief. It is important that they give themselves time to mourn their loss. A new pregnancy too close to an obstetric disaster can be started in a state of dread. They want to embark upon that pregnancy in anticipation and not in fear.

'What will happen in the next pregnancy?' The woman should be encouraged to book early for early should ultrasonography in a future pregnancy. Full hospital consultant antenatal care be offered, with ultrasound surveillance of the pregnancy for the couple's own reassurance. In the third trimester, a kick chart and CTGs are also reassuring. Admission should be offered to 'carry her over' the time of the past stillbirth, if that is thought to be appropriate. There is often a place for preterm delivery and even elective Caesarean section. The couple must feel confident in the obstetric service that will be offered in a future pregnancy.

Before their discharge from hospital, bereavement counselling must be offered to them. A contact number for the Stillbirth and Neonatal Death Society

(SANDS) should be given to them, as well as a copy of the Society's booklet *The loss of your baby*. The woman's own GP should be informed. Lactation will need to be suppressed. A 2-week course of bromocriptine 2.5 mg twice a day with food should be given. Arrangements are made for a subsequent follow-up appointment for postnatal examination and discussion of the post-mortem findings. This should not be at the end of an antenatal clinic, where the presence of vastly pregnant women may be upsetting.

It can be seen that a considerable amount of time needs to be given to such couples. It is worth while for the consultant's registrar or SHO to attend the pre-discharge session. Medical school, and indeed society, does not do much in training us to cope with grief. To be able to put an arm around a woman's shoulders and let her cry is so important and yet so simple. The doctor is not just there to give information counselling, but also to be involved in the counselling of their bereavement.

Neonatal death

The baby is born alive and transferred to the neonatal unit. The parents are aware of the baby's condition and to some degree are able to prepare and brace themselves for the grim event of their baby's death. Most neonatal units have facilities that will permit parents to stay on the unit and remain close to their baby. In addition to the normal follow-up described above for stillbirths, it is of value for the couple to see the paediatrician again at a later date.

Perinatal death checklist

 (1) allow parents to see and handle the baby;

 (2) provide polaroid photographs;

 (3) inform consultant obstetrician;

 (4) inform womans' GP;

 (5) notify community midwife;

 (6) medical photography and X-ray requested;

 (7) all other appropriate investigations performed;

 (8) consent for post-mortem given/refused;

 (9) religious needs of couple catered for;

(10) funeral arrangements discussed;

(11) pre-discharge consultation with senior member of the consultant team;

(12) postnatal visit arranged.

Maternal death

The international definition of maternal death is one which occurs during pregnancy and within 42 days following delivery.

'*Direct*' deaths result from obstetric complications during pregnancy, labour, and the puerperium.

'*Indirect*' deaths result from a pre-existing disease or one which developed during the pregnancy, such as diabetes.

'*Fortuitous*' deaths result from causes unrelated to the pregnancy, such as malignant disease and road traffic accidents.

'*Late*' deaths are those which occur after the 42-day limit but within a year of pregnancy. Many of these deaths will prove to be fortuitous but direct deaths will be included, such as those due to choriocarcinoma.

In the Report on Confidential Enquiries into Maternal Deaths in the UK (1988–90) there were 325 deaths reported to the Enquiry, 48 of which were late deaths. Excluding the late deaths, of the 227 remaining deaths 52 per cent (145) were direct, 34 per cent (93) indirect, and 14 per cent (39) fortuitous; 31 per cent (87) of the deaths occurred before 28 weeks' gestation. The direct maternal mortality rate of the constituent countries of the UK, ranged between 2.4 and 7.4 per 1 000 000 total births. This implies that in a large obstetric unit with 5000 deliveries per annum, there will be one maternal death every 2½ years.

The maternal mortality rate for 1988–90 was 7 per 100 000 maternities resulting in a livebirth or stillbirth. The true number would involve all pregnancies including spontaneous and induced terminations of pregnancy, as well as ectopics and live and stillbirths. This data is either unreliable or unobtainable.

The two major causes of maternal death are hypertensive disorders (18.6 per cent) and pulmonary embolism (16.6 per cent). These are followed by early pregnancy deaths from ectopic and abortion (16.5 per cent), haemorrhage (15.2 per cent), amniotic fluid embolism (7.6 per cent), sepsis (4.8 per cent), anaesthesia (2.8 per cent), and ruptured uterus (1.4 per cent). Other direct deaths together accounted for 16.6 per cent.

The Report has shown that in many instances there has been substandard care, not only on the part of medical services but also as a result of the actions of the woman and her family which will usually be beyond the control of clinicians. The inexperience of junior medical staff and midwives in an emergency situation repeatedly emerges as a factor in some maternal deaths. These deaths might have been avoidable had skilled assistance been sought earlier. The need for on-site high-dependency units and intensive care facilities is stressed.

When the disaster of maternal death occurs, it is a catastrophic experience for the family. It also has a devastating effect on the attending medical and midwifery staff. It is essential that the consultant on duty attends as an emergency to see the woman's partner and family and does everything possible to inform and support them at this dreadful time. It is also the consultant's role to give support to the medical and nursing staff. This is not the time to be judgemental. It is vital to ensure that the records are fully documented. There may be later medico-legal implications. The patient's GP must be informed immediately of the situation. A post-mortem will be required.

In the UK every maternal death must be informally notified to the district Director of Public Health. The enquiry form (MCW97) is then initiated and the Regional Assessors informed.

10   Postnatal period

The postnatal period, or puerperium, is defined as the time taken for the uterus to involute back to the normal non-pregnant size. This is usually 6 weeks postpartum.

Following delivery, the mother may experience a bout of quite violent shivering. She should be reassured that this is a completely normal reaction to the delivery. After any perineal repair is carried out, she is washed and prepared for transfer to the ward. All documentation is completed, including the case records and labour ward register.

Routine care

A significant number of women will seek to be discharged home to the care of their community midwife and GP within a few hours of delivery. This is usually because of the demands of a family at home who seem unable to cope without the presence of the mother. Unfortunately, this can mean that the woman who is most in need of postnatal rest is the one least likely to get it.

The standard routine observations that are carried out on return to the ward include initial pulse rate, blood pressure, and temperature readings. If these are normal, daily recordings of the pulse rate and temperature will be sufficient. In the event of there having been antenatal hypertension, 4-hourly blood pressure readings are continued.

It is important to check that urine output is adequate. It is very easy for urinary retention and subsequent overflow to develop in the early puerperium.

The fundal height of the uterus is checked daily to ensure that involution is occurring normally. The lochia are observed and the volume, colour, and odour are noted. Very offensive lochia will require further investigation. The woman is encouraged to care for her own perineum by using the bidet after each bowel movement.

The aims of postnatal care

- to establish a method of feeding
- to detect and treat any puerperal complications:
  infection
  thrombo-embolism
  secondary postpartum haemorrhage
  depression and related disorders
- to discuss future contraception.

Infant feeding

The decision as to whether or not to breast-feed is usually made antenatally by the majority of women. Antenatal clinics can offer the services of a skilled midwife to help and advise patients who are uncertain or concerned about a particular method of feeding. The advantages and disadvantages of breast- and bottle-feeding should be discussed so that the woman can make up her mind with full information. Some women find the thought of breast-feeding repellent. For others it is the ultimate fulfillment of being a mother. Among other advantages, 'bonding' is thought to be stronger in breast-fed babies.

Breast-feeding

The woman who intends to breast-feed her baby can do much to prepare for this antenatally. From 30 weeks the breasts should be gently massaged towards the nipples, which in turn should be gently rolled between finger and thumb. In this way, retracted nipples can be encouraged to protract, although it may be necessary to use Waller breast shells to overcome retraction. She should be taught how to manually express colostrum from the breasts and so clear milk ducts which the baby would otherwise have to do by feeding. This manoeuvre not only encourages the flow of colostrum but may prevent breast engorgement caused by thick colostrum. The skin over the nipples does not require any preparation apart from being kept clean. Techniques to 'harden' the nipples are unnecessary.

The sooner the baby is put to the breast the better. Considerable skill and reassurance are required to teach and encourage the first-time breast-feeder. She will need to be taught the most comfortable position to adopt while feeding and how to ensure that the baby is 'fixed' correctly to the areola around the nipple so as to avoid 'chewing' of the nipple. It is unusual for the woman who wants to breast-feed to be unable to do so. Difficulties tend to arise if the mother has not been taught correctly or is not particularly well motivated. Cracked, sore nipples or inverted nipples can also discourage mothers from persisting with breast-feeding.

Initially the flow of milk is low and only colostrum is secreted. This is assisted by the mother maintaining a good fluid intake.

> Breast-feeding is the best stimulant to encourage lactation.

Many mothers feed their babies 'on demand', building up to 10 minutes on each breast, allowing time for 'wind' to be burped spontaneously between sides. It is in the mother's sleep interests if feeds can be adjusted to a 3- to 4-hourly regimen.

If there are initial problems with feeding, there is the risk of breast engorgement. The use of a breast pump or manual expression of milk will relieve engorged breasts.

It is generally recommended that breast-feeding should continue for at least 3–4 months and many women will wish to breast-feed for considerably longer. In under-developed countries the advantages of long-term breast-feeding are considerable, because it is free and there is less risk of infant death from gastroenteritis resulting from poor hygiene in preparing bottle feeds. The high levels of IgA and antiviral agents in both colostrum and breast milk confer a passive immunity to the baby which can only be protective. Furthermore, artificial feeds may not be readily available and can involve considerable expense.

Contraindications to breast-feeding

- breast implant (breast augmentation)
- previous surgery for breast abscess
- maternal phenylketonuria
- drugs taken by mother:
  lithium
  cytotoxic drugs
  immunosuppressants
- baby with cleft palate
- active maternal tuberculosis
- very poor maternal health
- puerperal psychoses.

It is not always easy to be sure that the breast-fed baby is receiving sufficient milk. All babies will initially lose weight until lactation is fully established. The underfed baby will not gain weight satisfactorily and will cry excessively, often from thirst. Test-weighing the baby before and after feeds over a 24-hour period will indicate how much breast milk the baby is receiving. If necessary, supplementary feeds and occasionally even a change to bottle feeding may be required. After the first 2 weeks of breast-feeding it is very difficult to overfeed the baby.

Bottle-feeding ('artificial feeding')

It is essential that the mother who has decided to bottle-feed her baby is not made to feel guilty for not breast-feeding. This can only interfere with the enjoyment of caring for her baby and the 'bonding' process. Adequate time must be spent in teaching her how to prepare the bottle, select the right sized teat, and prepare the feed. She must be taught how to sterilize the bottles either by boiling or immersing in a dilute solution of hypochlorite (Milton).

> The importance of hygiene cannot be over-stressed. Gastroenteritis is still the major cause of infant death in the UK.

Bottle feeds are of high quality and mimic human breast milk as closely as possible. The cow's milk used in artificial feeds contains more protein (casein) and less sugar (lactulose) than found in human milk, while the fat content is similar. The higher level of casein tends to make cow's milk less digestible. The milk is fortified with additional iron and vitamins.

As with breast-feeding, bottle-feeding is generally 'on demand' and this should gradually settle to 3- to 4-hourly intervals. In time, it should be possible to miss out the late-night feed, thus allowing the parents to sleep through the night.

The volume of milk given commences at 20 ml/kg per day and builds up to 150 ml/kg per day by the seventh day. (For the non-metric mother, this is equivalent to $2\frac{1}{2}$ fl.oz./lb per day.)

Very occasionally, babies will exhibit an apparent allergy to cow's milk. A change from the cow's milk protein to soya milk resolves the problem.

Postnatal complications

Infection

A puerperal pyrexia is any febrile illness where the temperature is 38°C (100.4°F) or higher during the first 14 days postpartum.

Puerperal pyrexia is no longer a notifiable illness. However, this does not imply that the causes of pyrexia are now considered to be trivial.

Although the cause may seem obvious from the nature of the symptoms, a full examination is important. This will include examination of the breasts, chest, abdomen, perineum, and legs.

Investigations in all cases of puerperal pyrexia

(1) **mid-stream urine sample** for microscopy, organisms and culture;

(2) **cervical swab** for culture (a high vaginal swab is unsuitable for endometritis);

(3) **blood culture**;

(4) **sputum culture** (if obtainable).

Causes of puerperal pyrexia
- chest infection:
    post anaesthesia
- breast infection:
    mastitis
    breast abscess
- urinary tract infection:
    pyelonephritis
    cystitis
- genital tract infection:
    endometritis
    infected episiotomy or tear
- wound infection:
    wound abscess or cellulitis
- septicaemia
- deep vein thrombosis
- unrelated causes:
    appendicitis
    cholecystitis
    tonsilitis
    influenza.

Breast infection

Breast infection is generally a preventable condition if good lactation is maintained. Poor teaching of how to breast-feed correctly leads to sore or cracked nipples, breast engorgement, milk stasis, and eventually infection.

Breast engorgement is a relatively common finding by the third postnatal day. The mother may be pyrexial and complain of very hard, swollen, and tender breasts. This should not be mistaken for mastitis and is not an indication for antibiotic therapy. Milk should not be expressed at this stage as this is an excellent stimulus for further lactation. The breasts should be well supported with a well-fitting bra. Warm bathing of the breasts and analgesics are helpful. Fluid intake should be reduced. If the mother is very keen to continue to breast-feed, temporary reduction of lactation can be obtained by giving bromocriptine 2.5 mg twice daily for just 24 hours. When the breasts are more comfortable, milk can be expressed and breast-feeding can continue. If the mother does not wish to breast-feed, bromocriptine 2.5 mg twice daily with food (to avoid intense nausea) is continued for 14 days.

Mastitis is usually the result of *Staphylococcus aureus* gaining access to a lobe of breast tissue via a crack in the nipple. There may have been pre-existing duct stasis from thick colostrum which had not been expressed antenatally, as well as engorgement. The first sign of infection is maternal pyrexia. On examination, there is a reddened segment of the breast which is tender. The treatment at this early stage of breast infection is antibiotic therapy with flucloxacillin. Lactation should, at least temporarily, be suppressed.

Breast abscess is quite a rare complication of the puerperium as it is the result of inadequately treated mastitis. It generally occurs around the second postnatal week when the woman is already discharged from hospital. As a result, the obstetrician is often not even given the opportunity of treating this condition, since the majority of cases tend to be referred to the general surgeons. The mother may feel quite unwell with a febrile 'flu-like' illness. On examination, she will have a tender, swollen area on the breast. Brawny oedema of the skin is highly suggestive of an underlying abscess; a fluctuant swelling, if present, is the final confirmation.

> The surgical principle in the treatment of any abscess is drainage. *Do not* treat a breast abscess initially with antibiotics.

The inappropriate use of antibiotics for breast abscess will only lead to loculation of the abscess cavity, making subsequent successful drainage virtually impossible. Recurrent abscess formation and breast induration may result.

Surgical drainage is carried out under general anaesthesia. A small radial incision should be made over the abscess site. The size of the abscess cavity can be startlingly huge and contain copious quantities of pus. A swab of the pus is sent for culture. The cavity must be explored for any signs of loculation, which must also be drained. It is essential to drain the abscess cavity and a corrugated drain is ideal for this purpose. If the abscess is in an upper quadrant of the breast, dependent drainage is more difficult. To avoid subsequent loculation, it may be necessary to drain the cavity from below, placing the exit of the drain beneath the lower curvature of the breast so as to mask the exit scar. Antibiotic therapy with flucloxacillin can be commenced postoperatively. Lactation must be suppressed.

Urinary tract infection

Urinary tract infections are the commonest cause of puerperal pyrexia. Ureteric dilatation leads to urinary stasis and encourages ascending infection. Catheterization performed during labour or before Caesarean section may be a further predisposing factor.

This may be the woman's first urinary tract infecion, or she may have had recurring infections antenatally.

She may be asymptomatic, or she may have symptoms of pyelonephritis with rigors, nausea and vomiting, lower abdominal pain, and loin pain. A mid-stream urine sample, catheter sample, or a supra-pubic aspiration from the bladder will confirm the diagnosis. Microscopy of the urine will indicate the probability of a urinary tract infection by the white cell count. Treatment is the same for both pregnant and non-pregnant women. While awaiting the culture and sensitivities report, she should be commenced on appropriate antibiotic therapy. The commonest infecive agent is *E. coli*. Infections are also commonly due to *Streptococcus faecalis*, Proteus, and less frequently, Pseudomonas. It is important to check that the urine is clear on completion of the course of antibiotics.

In the case of recurrent antenatal infections, it would be very reasonable to maintain the woman on antibiotics for the duration of the pregnancy and puerperium. Intravenous urography should be deferred until 3 months postpartum so as to give time for the changes caused by pregnancy to disappear. Abnormalities such as renal staghorn calculi may be found.

Genital tract infection

Genital tract infections are a cause of maternal morbidity and mortality. In the Report on Confidential Enquiries into Maternal Deaths in the UK 1985–87, there were 17 direct deaths associated with genital tract sepsis. The infecting organisms were beta-haemolytic streptococci, *E. coli, Staphlococcus aureus, Enterobacter cloacae, Clostridium perfringens, Streptococcus millerii*, and anaerobes. In these deaths the onset of sepsis was usually insidious and rapidly fulminated. Disseminated intravascular coagulopathy was associated with two of the four streptococcal septicaemic deaths.

Predisposing factors for genital tract infection

- repeated vaginal examinations in labour (four or more) when membranes have ruptured
- prolonged premature rupture of membranes
- chorioamnionitis
- Caesarean section, episiotomy, vaginal and cervical tears
- retained placenta, membranes or clot.

Genital tract infection most commonly takes the form of an endometritis, although episiotomies and tears can also become infected. Infection may occur following a normal vaginal delivery, but is a significantly more frequent occurrence after Caesarean section. This is probably due to chorioamnionitis or ascending vaginal infection. A raw placental bed after delivery and the presence of an incision in the uterus provide an ideal environment for infection to gain a foothold. There is a definite place for the use of prophylactic antibiotic cover at Caesarean section in cases of prolonged labour or prolonged ruptured membranes (Cefuroxime 1.5 g or Augmentin 1.2 g intravenously, followed by further treatment if indicated).

On examination, the woman may appear to be very unwell, with a high temperature and tachycardia. The uterus may be bulky and tender.

> In fulminating infection the patient may remain afebrile, which can lead to delay in investigation and treatment.

In very severe cases, pelvic abscesses may form and even progress to peritonitis. There is usually an offensive, purulent vaginal discharge. A high vaginal swab is not a particularly helpful investigation owing to the presence of other contaminating organisms. A carefully taken cervical swab is more likely to provide an uncontaminated sample. There are techniques for obtaining transcervical samples from the endometrial cavity so as to further avoid contamination by vaginal organisms. A blood and urine culture should also be requested.

> Treatment of genital tract infection must be vigorous.

Broad-spectrum antibiotics must be given to cover both streptococcal and anaerobic infections such as bacteroides. It is recommended that the combination of amoxycillin-clavulanate (Augmentin), metronidazole, and either gentamycin or third-generation cephalosporin are used in combination. Once cultures and sensitivities have been obtained, the antibiotic therapy can be appropriately modified. Very occasionally, a pelvic abscess will need to be drained.

> In severe cases of pelvic sepsis do not hesitate to seek expert bacteriological advice.

A *wound abscess* can complicate Caesarean section. The patient presents with a swinging pyrexia and feels very hot and unwell. Drainage of an abscess must be encouraged. There is a place for hot kaolin poultices which are not only soothing but can also lead to spontaneous drainage of the abscess. A patient using a poultice should be warned that she may notice a sudden gush of highly offensive pus from the wound and should call for nursing assistance; she will, however, feel dramatically better. Sometimes it is necessary to surgically drain a wound abscess. This can be very successfully performed under local anaesthetic. There may be a need to open the entire incision line so as to adequately clean the wound of slough and encourage secondary healing by granulation. There are several different adsorbent agents which may be used to pack a wound so that it does not close over from above too soon and so leave an infected cavity beneath the skin.

If there is *cellulitis* around the abdominal wound, antibiotic therapy can be helpful. The infecting organism is usually staphyococcal and responds rapidly to flucloxacillin.

An *infected episiotomy* is often due to a poor surgical repair. It can be exquisitely tender and almost impossible for the patient to sit down at all. The suture line may appear to break down and if this occurs the process should be assisted, even if it means removing some of the suture material. The episiotomy wound can then be kept clean and will heal rapidly without secondary repair being required at all.

Septicaemia occasionally follows puerperal infection and may progress to *endotoxic* or *bacteraemic shock* (*Gram-negative shock*). Almost any infection can lead to shock, the commonest being the Gram-negative aerobic bacteria *E. coli* and Klebsiella, and the anaerobic *Bacteroides fragilis*. The Gram-positive bacteria include Streptococci, *Clostridium welchii*, and Staphyococci. Tachycardia, hypotension, and circulatory collapse follow. This is further complicated by disseminated intravascular coagulopathy (DIC). Vigorous intravenous antibiotic therapy with amoxycillin – clavulanate, metronidazole, and gentamycin – is indicated and combined with measures to support the circulation using Haemaccel, whole blood, and fresh frozen plasma (if DIC). The use of inotropic drugs such as dopamine and dobutamine by intravenous infusion will improve cardiac output and thereby improve tissue perfusion.

In cases of septic shock, the facility of an intensive care unit is essential.

Thrombo-embolism (both antenatal and postnatal)

In the Report on Confidential Enquiries into Maternal Deaths in the UK 1988–90, thrombo-embolism was the major cause of maternal death.

There were 33 deaths from thrombosis and/or thrombo-embolus, 24 from pulmonary embolism and 9 from cerebral thrombosis. There were 13 antenatal maternal deaths, 7 of which occurred before 20 weeks gestation and 11 before 33 weeks.

A clinical diagnosis of DVT was only made in 2 of the 13 antenatal deaths where autopsy subsequently revealed its presence.

There were 11 postnatal maternal deaths from resulting from pulmonary embolism. There were 3 vaginal deliveries and 8 Caesarean sections. Two-thirds of the deaths after Caesarean section occurred within 14 days of delivery. Two-thirds of the deaths after vaginal delivery occurred after 14 days.

Predisposing factors for thromo-embolism

- increasing maternal age
- past history of thrombo-embolism
- obesity
- Caesarean section
- immobilization (especially postoperatively)
- presence of lupus anticoagulant
- the use of oestrogen to suppress lactation.

Women with a past history of thrombo-embolism should receive prophylactic heparin therapy. Calcium heparin 5000 units twice daily is self-administered by the woman by subcutaneous injection. She must be taught how to give herself the injections correctly using pre-loaded syringes. Heparin assays are required every 1–2 weeks to ensure that the dosage is adequate. If low molecular weight heparin is to be used, a daily dosage of 5000 units subcutaneously is sufficient. The advantage of low molecular weight heparin at this dosage is that no screening of heparin levels is required. Heparin does not cross the placenta, whereas warfarin will do so and will anticoagulate the fetus. Apart from the interval between the onset of labour and 6 hours postpartum, heparin is given throughout the pregnancy and continued for 6 weeks postpartum.

Dieting is unlikely to be particularly beneficial in the obese woman during pregnancy. Her main risk of DVT will arise from any prolonged immobilization, especially linked to postoperative recovery. During Caesarean section, anti-thrombo-embolic stockings or pneumatic anti-thrombotic boots should be worn by the obese patient (and any other high-risk patient). Postoperatively, pro-phylactic heparin therapy should be given (which does not increase the risk of haemorrhage). An alternative for the high-risk patient who has no allergies, asthma, or cardiac or renal problem is to cover surgery with an infusion of dex-tran 70. Very rarely anaphylactic reactions may occur. No more than 1000 ml should be administered in any one infusion over a period of 6 hours. Dextran 70 and heparin must not be used together owing to a synergistic effect between them.

The classical signs of DVT are swelling of the leg and tenderness over the thrombus site. The woman complains of calf pain. The entire leg is swollen if the thrombosis involves the ilio-femoral veins. Unfortunately, the signs of throm-bosis are not always so clear-cut and are generally unreliable, especially in those cases involving the pelvic veins alone. Attempts to elicit Homan's sign as an aid to the diagnosis of DVT affecting the leg should be abandoned, as the manoeuvre itself has been known to actually cause pulmonary embolism. Confirmation of DYT by Doppler ultrasonic examination can be useful when there is a major DVT involving the ilio-femoral veins, as there will be an absence of the characteristic flow sounds over the femoral vein when the calf muscles are gently compressed. However, ultrasound is ineffective in diagnosing calf vein DVT. The antenatal diagnosis of DVT is made even more difficult if there is reluctance to carry out a venogram. The pregnancy can always be shielded with a lead apron. Obviously there are no problems in using venograms postnatally. Antenatal DVTs most commonly affect the left leg. There is an equal distribution postnatally.

DVT may be associated with a low grade pyrexia. In the puerperium this may be due to a septic pelvic vein thrombosis and may progress to pulmonary embolism. In such cases a combination of broad-spectrum antibiotic therapy as described for pelvic infection, and high-dose intravenous heparin is given to achieve urgent anticoagulation. An initial bolus loading dose of 5000 units is given, followed by a continuous infusion of 24 000–40 000 units per day by pump. The heparin activity is monitored by the activated partial thromboplastin time (PTTK) which should be between 1.5 and 3 times the control value. When the DVT has resolved, prophylactic subcutaneous heparin therapy 5000–10 000 units twice daily is continued until 6 weeks postpartum.

A venogram is of little help when there is an ilio-femoral thrombosis. A vena-cavagram is carried out via the femoral vein of the unaffected leg. If both legs are affected due to a thrombus involving the bifurcation of the inferior vena cava, then the jugular vein is used to demonstrate the extent of the thrombus. In this situation, there is occasionally an indication to insert an umbrella filter under local anaesthetic and image intensifier control.

Indications for insertion of a vena cava filter

- recurrent pulmonary emboli in spite of adequate anticoagulant therapy
- a large ilio-femoral thromosis with labour being imminent;
- when a vena-cavagram demonstrates that a portion of thrombus is about to break off and embolize.

The classical symptoms and signs of pulmonary embolism include chest pain, dyspnoea, haemoptysis, hyperventilation cyanosis, and shock. The apparent absence of signs of a DVT in spite of the presence of any of the above symptoms is the commonest reason for withholding anticoagulant therapy. The most frequently-made incorrect diagnosis is chest infection.

Every antenatal or postnatal patient complaining of pain in the leg or chest, or of sudden dyspnoea, must be regarded as having a DVT or pulmonary embolism until proven otherwise.

Isotope lung scans are safe in the third trimester. Pulmonary angiography may be necessary to confirm the diagnosis. Rapid diagnosis may be possible in future using MRI scans.

Urgent antibiotic and anticoagulant therapy is required. If there is reasonable evidence to suspect pulmonary embolism, it is justifiable to give a bolus dose of heparin and set up the heparin infusion, without awaiting absolute confirmation. Should subsequent investigation show that there was no embolism present, the heparin is simply discontinued.

Secondary postpartum haemorrhage (PPH)

Secondary PPH is defined as any significant bleeding from the genital tract occurring more than 24 hours after delivery.

The commonest causes of early secondary PPH are retained products of conception and retained clot. The products may only consist of a few fragments of placental tissue or membranes or may, surprisingly, be a very large portion of placenta. Late PPH is more likely to be associated with intrauterine infection whether or not there are retained products.

Secondary PPH is largely preventable by carefully checking that the membranes and placenta are complete at delivery. If there is any doubt as to the completeness of the third stage, exploration of the uterine cavity at that time is essential. It is especially embarrassing for the surgeon if a large portion of placenta is retained in the uterus after Caesarean section. It is important that the uterine cavity is briefly checked for retained placental remnants or membranes before closure of the incision.

Retained clot has the same effect as retained placental tissue. The most likely cause is blood which has not been adequately expressed from the uterus after the third stage of labour. Firm compression of the uterus at the end of a Caesarean section can prevent this problem occurring postoperatively. Good uterine contraction postpartum must be maintained in those clinical situations where primary PPH is more likely.

The uterus that contains retained products or clot tends to involute more slowly and remains larger than expected. There is a greater likelihood of endometritis and pelvic sepsis. Ultrasonography will confirm the presence of retained products and evacuation will then be indicated.

If there are already signs of infection, antibiotic therapy as described in pelvic sepsis should be initiated before evacuation is attempted. Great care must be taken at evacuation owing to the increased risk of uterine perforation. Heavy bleeding, even in the presence of infection, takes priority and must be controlled. Intravenous ergometrine 0.25 mg should be given. Blood may need to be cross-matched and given.

Many cases of secondary PPH occur once women have been discharged from hospital. Readmission of mother and baby (if she is breast-feeding) can cause problems for some gynaecological units that may not have facilities to care for a newborn baby. If bleeding has been heavy enough to warrant readmission, it is heavy enough to warrant exploration of the uterus. To keep the patient in hospital for a day or two 'to see if bleeding settles' is time-wasting and may be dangerous.

Depression and related problems

A woman will frequently experience swings in mood in the days following delivery. Initial anxiety in labour about her own well-being and that of her baby is followed by the 'high' of a successful delivery with a happy outcome. The 'fourth day blues' are well-recognized almost as a normal reaction to the earlier elation. In the majority of cases, simple reassurance that her apparent depression is very common and will pass quickly is all the treatment that will be required.

Occasionally, depression becomes an increasing feature of the puerperium and of the months that follow. Weeping, irritability, insomnia, tiredness, and even loss of interest in the baby and her family are symptoms that must be taken seriously by nursing and medical attendants. Reassurance, advice, and close support is essential. Treatment with antidepressant drugs under close supervision may be necessary to prevent the more serious sequelae of depression which can include infanticide and even suicide. Psychiatric assistance may be necessary. It is usually possible to admit both mother and baby to a psychiatric unit.

Puerperal psychosis will affect 1 in 1000 patients. Auditory hallucinations, delusions, and bizarre behaviour are the characteristic features. Urgent referral for admission to a psychiatric unit is essential.

Contraceptive advice

For many women, the prospect of ever having intercourse again, especially if coping with a tender episiotomy, is something they would prefer not to think about at all! It is quite normal for the postnatal woman's libido to be very low on returning home. Tiredness due to disturbed nights and associated depression will not do much to restore her interest in sex.

One of the chief roles of postnatal care is to make certain that future contraception is discussed, ideally before the woman is discharged from hospital.

Some patients will require intramuscular progestagen (Depo-Provera 150 mg) to give absolute contraception in order to cover a rubella vaccination, or to provide interim contraception while awaiting an IUCD insertion.

The combined oral contraceptive Pill is not contraindicated for breast-feeding mothers and does not, in fact, suppress lactation. However, its use should be deferred until after the puerperium to reduce the risk of DVT. In the meantime, the use of barrier methods such as the condom should be advised.

If the cap had been used before the current pregnancy, the woman must be advised not to rely upon the old cap but be fitted with a new one after the puerperium.

An alternative for many women would be to commence the progesterone-only Pill immediately.

Most women know that breast-feeding in itself cannot be relied upon as a method of contraception, but it is best to make sure that she is aware of this.

The 'withdrawal method' of contraception should be discouraged as a reliable method of contraception.

The woman must be happy that she is going to use a method of contraception that will suit her and her partner and is one in which she has confidence. There is no need for her to wait for her postnatal visit before resuming intercourse.

Puerperal sterilization may have been requested during the antenatal period (see p. 53).

Pre-discharge postnatal check

Every woman requires to be seen and checked before her discharge from hospital. She must be feeling well in herself and all nursing observations should be normal. She must be afebrile with a normal pulse and blood pressure. On examination, the fundus of the uterus must be involuting well and there must be no uterine tenderness. By day one the uterus should be 24 weeks in size, by day five 16 weeks, and by day ten it is no longer palpable per abdomen. A Caesarean section scar or episiotomy must be healing without problem.

A feeding method must be established. A woman should not go home both breast-feeding and giving supplementary feeds.

Contraception must be discussed. Finally, ask her if there are any problems that she would like to discuss.

The community midwife is informed of the patient's discharge so that postnatal observation of her and her baby may continue. It is important that the Guthrie test is carried out, if not already performed in hospital (p. 237).

Postnatal visit

This visit takes place 6 weeks after delivery at the end of the puerperium. If there have been complex problems antenatally or in labour, this final postnatal check is usually at the consultant unit. Uncomplicated pregnancies are followed up by the GP and community midwife.

The postnatal visit is really an opportunity to ensure that mother and baby are thriving and that there are no unresolved problems. The method of feeding is discussed and the weight gain of the baby is checked. The return of menstruation is enquired after.

The mother is then examined. She is weighed and her blood pressure is checked. The abdomen is palpated, the perineum is checked, and a gentle bimanual palpation is performed. The tenderness of any perineal repair is assessed and this is an appropriate time to enquire after any problems relating to intercourse.

The uterus should now have returned to the normal non-pregnant size.

If a cervical smear is required, it is best to defer this to 3 months postpartum.

Contraception is discussed. Unless sterilized in the puerperium, or unless there are unusual circumstances such as a donor insemination pregnancy, she must be made aware that she can now become pregnant again if contraceptive precautions are not taken. Further contraceptive advice may be necessary. The timing of any future pregnancy should be discussed.

Special precautions in a future pregnancy and, in particular, management plans are discussed at this time. It is very important that the mother knows of any potential problems in a future pregnancy. For example, if antenatal admission is going to be likely, she now has a young baby at home. It is particularly important that in any future pregnancy she books in to her GP surgery early, so that early referral can be made.

11   The DRCOG examination

The new format of the examination for the Diploma of the Royal College of Obstetricians and Gynaecologists (DRCOG) is not only a very thorough assessment of your knowledge and of the skills you have gained through experience, but also of your ability to apply what you know to different clinical situations as met in General Practice. A pass in the DRCOG is a recognition of your particular interest in the subject without being a specialist qualification.

Knowledge at an undergraduate level (MB) will not be sufficient to pass the DRCOG examination.

Requirements

The sole requirement is for a fully registered medical practitioner to have completed a specifically recognized 6 month combined post in obstetrics and gynaecology. (There is no additional requirement of attendance at family planning clinics although it is expected that all candidates will have the same theoretical knowledge that is required by doctors who wish to take the Diploma of the Faculty of Family Planning and Reproductive Health Care of the RCOG.) Full regulations, details, and the syllabus of the DRCOG examination are available from:

The Examination Secretary
The Royal College of Obstetricians and Gynaecologists
27 Sussex Place
London NW1 4RG
(Telephone: (0171) 262 5425 Fax (0171) 723 0575)

The DRCOG examination is held each April and October.

Format of the examination

The format of the examination changed radically in 1994.
The DRCOG now comprises:

- a multiple choice question (MCQ) paper
- an objective structured clinical examination (OSCE).

Obstetrics

A good general knowledge of obstetrics is essential. Particular emphasis is placed upon a clear understanding of the principles of preconceptual, antenatal, intranatal, and postnatal care, with the ability to recognize and manage the obstetric problems and emergencies that may arise.

Gynaecology

You are not expected to have an in-depth knowledge of how to carry out complex operative procedures. However, you must have a clear understanding of the investigation, diagnosis, and management of all general gynaecological disorders including the problems of genitourinary medicine and family planning. Particular attention is paid to the GP management of clinical situations as presented in the surgery.

Tips on DRCOG

There is no doubt that it is best to take the examination as soon as possible after fulfilling the necessary requirements. This usually means that it will be sat within 6 months of completing a DRCOG-recognized SHO post in obstetrics and gynaecology. If it is your intention to take the DRCOG, revision goes hand in hand with the post. It may otherwise be difficult to revise when you are in another post and working full time. Reading is essential but you will fail if you only know lists of facts. The OSCE in particular will test your practical ability, your competence in discussing a problem succinctly as well as your communication and counselling skills.

There are DRCOG courses that can give a very thorough grounding on the examination's requirements. However, if you have completed a good SHO post, you will have received feedback from your peers, midwives, registrars, senior registrars, and consultants. You will have regularly attended ward rounds, case presentations, seminars, lectures, perinatal mortality/morbidity meetings and postgraduate meetings. You will have had the opportunity to present topics, cases, or projects yourself, become involved in a journal club and maybe even research. Additional in-depth reading to consolidate your own clinical experience and some examination practice are all that is required to see you through the DRCOG.

Method of marking

You must pass both the MCQ paper and the OSCE to be awarded the DRCOG. The pass mark of each of these two parts is in fact very generous and should not pose a problem for the well-prepared candidate. The pass mark for each part of the examination is the mean score minus one standard deviation.

Multiple choice question (MCQ) paper

The MCQ paper lasts for 2 hours and tests your ability to remember facts relating to obstetrics, gynaecoloqy, and related subjects. The paper consists of 60 questions, each having five parts, totalling 300 questions. Each question consists of an initial statement followed by five numbered items. You will be required to answer on a computer answer sheet whether you know a particular item is TRUE or FALSE. One mark will be gained for every correct true or false answer. **DO NOT LEAVE AN ITEM BLANK.** Firstly, any mark on the paper such as a unclean erasure may be misinterpreted by the computer's optical scanner. Secondly, **there is no negative marking** which means that you will not be penalized for an incorrect answer. If you do not know the answer it is worth while to make an educated guess—you have a 50–50 chance of getting it right and gaining a mark. If your guess is incorrect you are not penalized.

MCQs are a very searching way of assessing knowledge, and a good technique and practice in answering this form of questioning is essential.

The objective structured clinical examination (OSCE)

The OSCE has replaced the previous clinical and oral examinations, having been shown to be a more valid and reliable method of testing relevant subjects. You will be asked to carry out day-to-day tasks that are based on your clinical exerience. You will be assessed on your ability to remember facts, interpret data, and solve problems. Your communication skills will be judged on how you interact with a 'role play' patient or an examiner. Because all of the candidates sitting the examination will be taking the same OSCE, there will be common standards for all.

The OSCE may be a new style of examination for you, although it is featuring more frequently now in undergraduate examinations. Detailed explanatory notes are available from the Royal College of Obstetricians and Gynaecologists. A video explaining the OSCE is held by all RCOG District Tutors and RCOG Regional Advisers.

The OSCE is held in several different venues in the UK, all the candidates being examined on the same day. Every OSCE centre has several identical *circuits* each of 22 *stations*. In order to process the number of candidates, there is a morning group and an afternoon group of candidates at each centre. The afternoon group will be quarantined in the centre's holding area by midday so that there can be no contact between the morning and afternoon groups once the examination has started. The morning group will leave the centre by a different exit so that there can be no communication with the afternoon candidates.

Reception area

On your arrival at the rception area of the centre, you will be welcomed and directed to the holding area.

Holding area

Here registration takes place, checking your candidate number, identification, *circuit number*, and *starting station number*. Seating, refreshments (non-alcoholic!), and toilet facilities are available. When all the candidates are assembled, a briefing of the examination is given by the Senior Examiner. There are also poster demonstrations on the style of the OSCE including an example question, and an opportunity to see the video.

Forty-five minutes before the examination, the candidates who are now in groups of 22 according to their circuit numbers, are moved in circuit number order by stewards to the marshalling area adjacent to the examination hall.

Marshalling area

You now stay in the marshalling area for your particular circuit. Coats and bags must be left here. Your circuit steward again checks that you know your station number and gives a final rebriefing.

Twenty minutes before the examination begins, each steward in turn takes his 22 candidates to the correct circuit.

Each circuit contains 22 stations or tables arranged in a hollow square or rectangle. Your steward checks that you are seated at the correct station and that your answer book commences with the top answer sheet matching your station number. The pack of answer sheets has already been labelled and sorted in the correct number sequence so that you will have your starting station at the top of the pack. For example, if you are seated at station number 6, the top sheet of your answer book will be the answer sheet for station 6.

You will be given a 5-minute warning and then a 1-minute warning before the examination commences.

The OSCE

At each station except two (see below) you will be asked to complete a task. The tasks will include answering structured written factual questions, problem solving from case histories or a video, and interpretation of information from test results. There may be a simulator or equipment which you will be expected to use correctly. There will also be interactive stations. Your answers to the questions or tasks set at each station mean that you will 'write', 'do', or 'speak'.

You will have 6 minutes at each station. This does not sound very long but it is in fact ample time. When the bell sounds after 6 minutes YOU MUST STOP WRITING IMMEDIATELY. You *move in a clockwise direction* (to avoid utter chaos!) to the next station *taking your answer book with you*.

You will be directed to leave each answer sheet in a collection tray.

In this way you cover all 22 stations regardless of your original point of entry into the circuit. So if your entry point was at station 6, you will continue clockwise to station 22 and then stations 1–5 to complete the 22 stations.

Two of the 22 stations are *rest stations* where you have no allotted task to carry out. If you become desperate to visit the toilet, it is very much in your interests to hold on until you reach a rest station so as not to miss out on scoring marks at a task station.

The *interactive stations* test your communication skills. You will be given information to read concerning the 'role play' patient (who is very well-briefed and well-informed) You will be marked on this station by both the examiner (who is only an observer) *and the 'patient' herself*. The mark given will depend upon the key points you discuss with her. Your communication skills are assessed by observing:

eye contact with the patient;
how you put the patient at ease;
avoiding medical jargon;
the patient's understanding of the problem;
how you listened to the patient;
how you picked up non-verbal signals (distress, etc.);
the offering of additional informationm that the patient would find helpful;
how follow-up was arranged.

The patient will mark you on how reassured she is by the way you have presented the information to her. In other words, whether she would ever want to see you again for a medical problem!

There are currently no stations that you *must* pass in order to pass the OSCE, although this may change in future examinations for the DRCOG. Therefore, at present you do not have to pass each station. ANSWER ALL THE QUEST-IONS. As there is no negative marking you will not be penalized for an incorrect answer.

The Senior Examiner will announce the start of the final (22nd) station. At the end of that 6 minutes you will be asked to stop writing. Remain seated until you are told to leave. Each circuit will then be escorted by its steward to the marshalling area. After collecting coats and bags you leave the centre by another exit. The morning group of candidates are thereby unable to communicate with the afternoon group who are already in the holding area.

The DRCOG is generally regarded as a very fair examination. It is a diploma worth holding, as a pass in the DRCOG is really giving a 'seal of approval' of your competence to undertake the practice of obstetrics and gynaecology within the setting of primary health care.

GOOD LUCK!

12   Obstetric history-taking and examination

In addition to a written examination and/or OSCE, medical schools will often require their students to sit a clinical and oral examination at the end of their undergraduate attachment in Obstetrics and Gynaecology. Although these do not now feature as part of the Diploma of the Royal College of Obstetricians and Gynaecologists (DRCOG), it is still a requirement for the higher Diploma of Membership of the RCOG (MRCOG).

I felt that it would be helpful to student readers if I devoted a section of the book to this aspect of their final exams.

The clinical examination

This essentially should be regarded as the antenatal clinic or surgery where you meet a new obstetric patient for the first time. Only this time it is as if the notes are mislaid and you have to take a history from scratch. You will have done this many times before, admitting patients to the ward or labour ward. So why panic?

To prepare for this you must practise taking obstetric histories as if for the exam itself. There is no doubt that it is far easier if you can prepare for the exam with a colleague and present histories to each other.

There is little point in staying up late revising the night before the clinical examination. Sleep is of more value to you. On the next day you will need to have your wits about you, not because there is going to be a trap laid for you, but simply so you can think clearly and have a good command of the knowledge that you undoubtedly have.

Give yourself plenty of time to get to the hospital where the exam is to be held, so that you arrive on time. Arriving in a rush or being late can only be an unnerving experience. Do not forget that your university finals is a professional exam. Look tidy and clean.

(The time allowed for taking the history and carrying out the examination will vary from centre to centre, but 30 minutes is an average time allocated, with an additional 15 minutes with the examiners. You may find that one of a pair of examiners is in attendance while you take the history and examine the patient. This can actually work in your favour, especially if the patient is a poor historian.)

You will be directed to a room or part of a ward to meet your patient. You will be given a clipboard and paper on which to write your history and examination findings. Introduce yourself to the patient. Shake hands.

In my role as an examiner, I have found that the quality of history-taking and presentation can vary considerably. By now you will have developed a method of taking and presenting an obstetric history. Make sure that the method you use is foolproof and does not leave any major gaps. The way in which you take the history is not necessarily the way in which you will present it. You will obtain some information that may not be relevant to present in the history but which you will have available if it is requested of you. The scheme I have outlined below is the one I use myself and it works for me!

The obstetric history

Make out a list of headings such as those below that you can tick off as you go along.

Name and age:

Obtain social details:
- married or single?
- age of her partner?
- how long together? are they still together?
- her occupation
- partner's occupation
- does she smoke? how much?
- does she indulge in alcohol? how much?

Past medical and surgical history:
- any serious illnesses or operations? (*If none ask 'Have you ever been admitted to hospital for anything?'*)
- any regular medications?
- any allergies?
- has she ever had a blood transfusion? if yes, why?
- does she know her blood group?

Past family history
- any serious illnesses among other members of the family?
- enquire specifically after diabetes, hypertension, TB.
- are there any children born to members of the family who are handicapped in any way, either physically or mentally?

Past obstetric history
- how many previous pregnancies have there been?

(*Enquire after each pregnancy in chronological order; go through the details of each pregnancy in a logical and progressive manner, i.e. start at the beginning*):
- year of pregnancy?
- place delivered?
- antenatal problems?
- duration of pregnancy? was labour spontaneous/induced? if induced, why?

- hours in labour?
- problems in labour?
- method of delivery? if forceps or Caesarean section, why?
- third stage complications?
- outcome of delivery; sex, weight, feeding method, alive and well?
- if a miscarriage, was she admitted? was evacuation of uterus performed? if termination of pregnancy, why?
- if rhesus-negative, did she receive anti-D after delivery, miscarriage, termination?

(*The advantage of taking the history this way is that you now have the foundations for the current pregnancy. There can be no nasty surprises. If you start the history with enquiry into the current pregnancy and she informs you about pain in her Caesarean section scar, that is an event you don't even know about and it may be unsettling in the exam environment*).

Current pregnancy
- was this pregnancy planned?
- how long trying? (*if this is her first pregnancy after trying for many years, ask after infertility investigations and treatment if not already known*)
- contraception prior to current pregnancy;
- were her periods regular? how often? how many days bleeding?

To establish her dates:
- date of last period?
- did it come when expected?
- was it a normal period?

(*Work out the EDD. Use an obstetric calculator if you wish. Check with the patient that the date you have reached agrees with what she thinks is her EDD. Work out the weeks of pregnancy reached. Does she agree with the number of weeks?*)

- any problems in early pregnancy such as bleeding, excessive vomiting?
- how many weeks pregnant when she first booked into hospital ANC?
- did she have a booking scan? did it agree with her dates? any problems found?
- did she have any special screening test for Down's syndrome and spina bifida? does she know the results?
- any further scans? detailed anomaly scan?
- when did she first feel movements?
- frequency of visits to GP/hospital;
- any additional tests?
- any problems as pregnancy progressed?
- any bowel or bladder problems?
- any bleeding?
- has she been given a kick chart? is she feeling adequate movements?
- is she feeling well?
- is she still working?

- is she on any medicines during the pregnancy?
- is she taking iron and folic acid tablets? at how many weeks did she start them?

(It is perfectly reasonable to ask her if any plans have been made for induction or delivery. Has she been told how the rest of the pregnancy is to be managed? Are there any special plans for her management in labour? How does she intend to feed the baby? YOU ARE CERTAIN TO BE ASKED 'How would you manage Mrs Smith's care?')

This may seem a formidable list of questions but it should not take more than 10 minutes to get through them. There is time to spend another few minutes just going through the relevant points in the history with the patient: *'You are Mrs Smith and this is your fourth baby . . .'*

There is no point in going through a detailed systems review. If you have obtained a history of hypertension in the current pregnancy it is then correct to enquire in greater depth into possible problems, such as headaches, visual disturbances, epigastric pain, special investigations, etc.

You now need to examine your patient. While doing so, you can go over any aspects of the history with her. You should also now be beginning to think out the opening statement in your presentation of the history to the examiners, which should take the form of a one-sentence summary.

Remember to have a nurse with you during the examination of the patient.

Ask if there is a urine sample to test for protein and sugar. If not, don't worry; you can at least say you asked.

General examination:

- assessment of general appearance, e.g. very petite, short stature, overweight, etc; ask for her height and weight
- check for anaemia
- check for peripheral oedema:

     pre-tibial *(pre-tibial over the medial aspect of the tibia, not over the fleshy lateral aspect; remember she has two legs! Examiners like to ask you, to demonstrate how you assess ankle oedema)*

     fingers *(has she had to remove rings?)*
     sacral area *(only if on prolonged bed rest)*
     abdominal wall *(persistent depression from fetal stethoscope)*;
     face *(ask her).*

Cardiovascular and respiratory systems: (BRIEFLY)

- pulse and blood pressure *(take BP to nearest 5 mm — 120/85 not 122/84)*; if obese? large cuff available, but don't waste time
- auscultate heart sounds; note any murmurs
- auscultate the chest
     included here:
- four-quadrant examination of the breasts.

Abdominal examination:

(*Depending upon your medical school, you may be able to treat this as a practice run to be repeated for the examiners when you present the case history.*)

OBSERVATION FINDINGS:

- distended abdomen; a very broad shape may suggest transverse lie; a flat plateau over the umbilicus may indicate OP position
- striae gravidarum old and new
- linea nigra
- operation scars (*look for laparoscopy scar*)
- fetal movements seen?

PALPATION OF THE ABDOMEN:

- fundal height (*use a tape-measure if you wish, to measure symphysio-fundal height; cm = weeks approx.*) uterine size should be compatible with, large, or small for dates;
- liquor volume; adequate, increased, or reduced
- lie (longitudinal, oblique, or transverse)
- presenting part; cephalic, breech or difficult to assess if very obese
- engaged? fifths palpable above the brim if cephalic (don't use fifths for a breech)
- position; LOA, OP, etc; (it is easier to hear FH through fetal back)
- auscultate FH for 10 seconds ($\times 6$ = rate) (*feel for patient's radial pulse at same time so as to determine that it is not the maternal pulse that is heard*).

This can all be accomplished within your allocated 30 minutes. If you have time, sort out how you will present the history. Try to spot the key topics arising from her history.

Two examiners now enter the room. One examiner asks the questions while the other listens. You will be asked to present a relevant history about the patient.

Presentation example:

This is Mrs Eunice Smith, who is 34 years of age and is now 36 weeks pregnant in her fourth pregnancy, her only previous baby having been delivered by emergency Caesarean section.

Mrs Smith is a housewife. Her husband has unfortunately been made redundant, having worked in a local building merchants. They own their house.

Mrs Smith stopped smoking when she found out that she was pregnant. She very occasionally has an alcoholic drink.

There is no relevant past medical or surgical history apart from that relating to her past obstetric history. Mrs Smith did not know her blood group but is sure that she is rhesus-positive. She had a 2-pint blood transfusion following her Caesarean section in her last pregnancy.

In the family history, her mother was a twin. She also has a first cousin (her mother's twin sister's child) who has Down' syndrome.

Mrs Smith has a significant past obstetric history:

Her first pregnancy was in 1988. At 12 weeks she bled heavily and required to be admitted to hospital. A scan showed that she had an incomplete abortion. She had an evacuation of retained products of conception.

In 1989, at 6 weeks' gestation she miscarried at home and did not require to be admitted to hospital.

In 1991 she became pregnant for the third time. This pregnancy progressed well until 32 weeks. An earlier scan had suggested that the placenta was covering the internal os of the cervix and this was confirmed as still being the case at 32 weeks. In view of the diagnosis of placenta praevia, she was admitted to the ward, so as to be in the safest environment should any bleeding occur. At 34 weeks she had a sudden APH in bed in the middle of the night and was transferred to the labour ward. The bleeding settled down and 24 hours later she was transferred back to the ward. She had two further transfers to the labour ward in the next 2 weeks. On the third occasion the bleeding did not settle and she was advised to have a Caesarean section. This was performed under general anaesthetic. She had a little boy weighing 6 lbs 1 oz. who was born in good condition. Mrs Smith had a 2-pint blood transfusion after delivery. She tried to breast-feed but found it very difficult as she had a lot of pain with her wound. She had to give up and bottle-feed instead.

This now brings us to her current pregnancy:

Her periods were always very regular, occurring every 28–30 days and lasting for 5 days. After her Caesarean section, she went onto the Pill for about 9 months. On stopping the Pill her periods rapidly settled down to their previous pattern.

Her last menstrual period began on 17 August 1994. This was a normal period, coming when it was expected and lasting the normal length of time. It was not a Pill-withdrawal bleed. This would give her an expected date of delivery of 24 May 1995 making her now just over 36 weeks pregnant by dates.

During this pregnancy she has been very well. There has not been any bleeding in early pregnancy, or since then.

She first booked into the antenatal at 10 weeks. A booking scan agreed with her dates.

At 15 weeks she had the local screening blood test carried out and was told that her risk of Down's syndrome was very remote. She did not wish to have an amniocentesis done, even though there is the family history of this condition.

At 18 weeks she had what sounds like a detailed scan. The size of the baby and the scan were still in agreement. No abnormality was seen in the baby. Mrs Smith was relieved to learn that the placenta was at the fundus of the uterus.

Antenatal care has been shared between the hospital and the GP. At 20 weeks Mrs Smith started on Pregaday, 1 tablet daily.

At 28 weeks Mrs Smith returned to the consultant antenatal clinic. All was well. She was asked to keep a mental check on fetal movements before commencing a kick chart at 32 weeks. She has always felt her ten movements by mid-morning.

Mrs Smith is now 36 weeks pregnant and very well. The method of delivery has not yet been decided, but she would prefer a Caesarean section.

So in summary, Mrs Smith is a 34-year-old gravida 4 para 1, her previous baby being delivered by emergency Caesarean section for placenta praevia; she is now 36 weeks pregnant, but no decision has yet been taken regarding the method of delivery.

You will now be asked whether or not you have examined Mrs Smith. You will be asked to present either your general findings, or any abnormal features found on general examination.

You may be asked to demonstrate any abnormal finding such as ankle oedema.

You will be invited to demonstrate your examination of the abdomen and give a running commentary as you do so. First of all, ask the patient to lie down comfortably with her arms by her side. The abdomen should be revealed from xiphisternum to pubis. Comment on your visual findings first *without touching the abdomen*:

> The abdomen is distended and compatible with pregnancy. There are a few old striae gravidarum and a faintly pigmented linea nigra. She has a scar from the Pfannenstiel incision for her Caesarean section. There are no other scars visible. I cannot see any fetal movements at present, although I did see movements at my earlier examination.
>
> On palpation (*demonstrate all aspects of the examination and don't rush it!*), the size of the uterus is compatible with dates. I am now measuring the fundal height from the top of the symphysis pubis to the fundus of the uterus, and it is 37 cm. The lie is longitudinal. The presentation is cephalic. The head is four-fifths palpable above the pelvic brim. The baby is in a left occipito-lateral position with the back along the left side of the uterus. The fetal heart is clearly heard through the baby's back. The rate before was 132 per minute.

Further questions may now take place while with the patient, before you all go to another room for in-depth questioning. **Remember to thank the patient for the help.**

You will probably have another 10–15 minutes with your examiners. Sit comfortably. Try to look interested and alert.

The examiners may now ask you any questions they wish, relating to the patient you have just examined.

For this patient the key questions will be:

- diagnosis of placenta praevia
- management of placenta praevia
- screening tests for Down's syndrome
- monitoring of fetal well-being
- plan of management:

    'How do you think this patient should be delivered and why?'

    'If you are contemplating a vaginal delivery, are there any investigations you would wish to carry out before reaching a decision?'

    'How would you manage her in labour?'

    'If you decided to carry out a Caesarean section and she asked you to sterilize her at the same time, how would you advise her?

Answer all questions as simply as a clearly as possible. Again, remember that there are no traps being set for you. Any traps are of your own making if your answers get bogged down in small-print that you really know nothing about.

After the clinical examination, go for a walk, get some fresh air, and above all have some lunch before the afternoon oral examination.

Oral examination

(This is usually split into 10 minutes with each examiner covering both obstetrics and gynaecology)
Try to appear confident and alert as you are called in to the oral examination. Sit comfortably. Your examiners are usually in a good mood, having been excellently fed by the host hospital.

This part of the examination can cover *any* aspect of your syllabus. Make sure that you can talk about the items that are commonly scattered upon the examiners' table between you and them. These include CTG traces, an amnihook, a doll and pelvis to demonstrate the mechanism of labour, a fetal skull and obstetric forceps. An IUCD may be dangled before you, as well as packets of the contraceptive pill.

If you are asked a question that you know absolutely nothing about, it is best to say so, rather than waffle and guess. If your examiners wish to chat between themselves discussing their own experiences of the topic in question, let them! It leaves less time for them to question you!

Recommended reading

Al-Azzawi, F. (1990). *A colour atlas of childbirth and obstetric techniques*. Wolfe Publishing,

Beischer, N. A. and Mackay, E. V. (1988). *Obstetrics and the newborn*, (2nd British edn). Bailliere Tindall,

Chamberlain, G. (1992). *ABC of antenatal care*. BMJ publication.

Gibb, D. M. F. (1991). *Common obstetric emergencies*. Butterworth-Heinemann,

Jarvis, G.J. (1994). *Obstetrics and gynaecology. A critical approach to clinical problems*. Oxford University Press.

Kaye, P. (1988). *Notes for the DRCOG*. Churchill Livingstone,

Liu, D. T. Y. and Fairweather, D. V. I. (1991). *Labour ward manual*. (2nd edn). Butterworths,

Llewellyn-Jones, D. (1991). *Fundamentals of obstetrics and gynaecology*, Vol. 1 Obstetrics (5th edn.). Faber and Faber,

Report on confidential enquiries into maternal depths in the United Kingdom 1988–90. HMSO, London.

May, A. (1994). *Epidurals for childbirth*. Oxford Univeristy Press.

Turnbull, A. and Chamberlain, G. (eds) (1989). *Obstetrics*. Churchill Livingstone, (Major reference source)

Wood, P. and Dobbie, H. G. (1989). *Electronic fetal heart rate monitoring: a practice guide*. Macmillan,

Index